CULINARY ESSENTIALS

Lab Manual

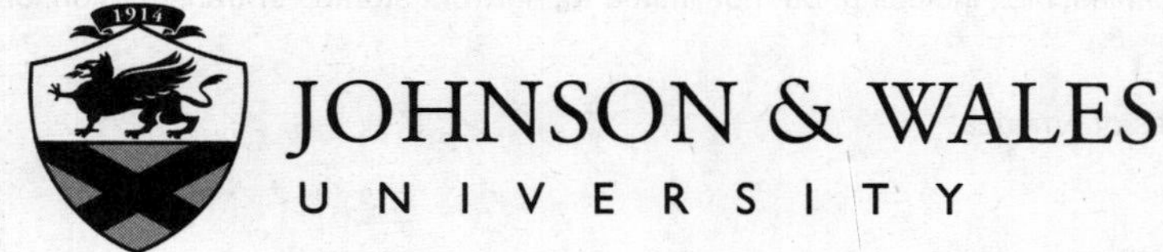

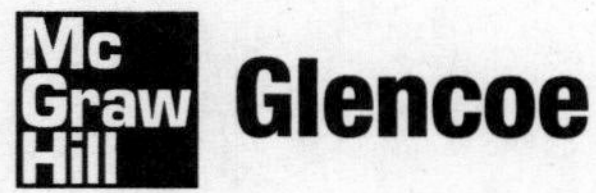

Contributors

Paul J. McVety Ed.D., Dean, Culinary Academics, Johnson & Wales University
Bradley J. Ware Ph.D., Professor, College of Culinary Arts, Johnson & Wales University
Deb Bettencourt, Special Projects Coordinator, College of Culinary Arts, Johnson & Wales University
John Chiaro, M.S., CEC, CCE, AAC, Associate Professor, College of Culinary Arts, Johnson & Wales University

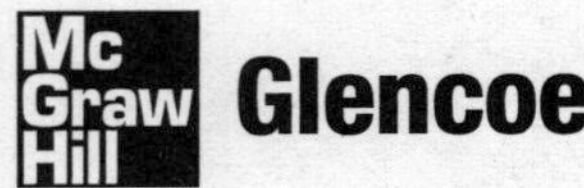

The McGraw·Hill Companies

Printed in the United States of America.

Send all inquiries to:
Glencoe/McGraw-Hill
21600 Oxnard Street, Suite 500
Woodland Hills, CA 91387

ISBN: 978-0-07-888442-9 (SE Lab Manual)
MHID: 0-07-888442-X (SE Lab Manual)

ISBN: 978-0-07-888443-6 (IAE Lab Manual)
MHID: 0-07-888443-8 (IAE Lab Manual)

2 3 4 5 6 7 8 9 066 14 13 12 11 10 09

Contents

Table of Contents

Chapter 1 Safety and Sanitation Principles

Section 1.1 Safety Basics

Science Project—Describe Sanitation Products....... 9

Section 1.2 Sanitation Challenges

Science Project—List Potential Hazards................ 10

Study Skills—Preparing a Place to Study 11

Certification Test Practice—Preparing for Tests...... 12

Content and Academic Vocabulary........................ 13

Culinary Review—Create a Fire Safety Plan 14

Chapter 2 HACCP Applications

Section 2.1 The Safe Foodhandler

Culinary Skills Project—Determining Foodhandler Dress Codes.. 17

Section 2.2 The HACCP System

Mathematics Project—Calculate Bacteria Growth 18

Section 2.3 The Flow of Food

Culinary Skills Project—Identify Contamination Hazards.. 19

Study Skills—Learning New Material.................. 20

Certification Test Practice—What to Ask Before a Test 21

Content and Academic Vocabulary...................... 22

Culinary Review—Measure Temperature Correctly.. 23

Unit 1 Culinary Safety

Competitive Events Practice—Make a Salad......... 26

Chapter 3 Foodservice Career Options

Section 3.1 Careers in Foodservice

English Language Arts Project—Develop a Career Plan.. 28

Section 3.2 Foodservice Trends

Social Studies Project—Track Trends 29

Section 3.3 Entrepreneurship

Mathematics Project—Determine Franchise Fees 30

Study Skills—Managing Study Time................... 31

Certification Test Practice—Taking True/False Tests.. 32

Content and Academic Vocabulary..................... 33

Culinary Review—Plan a Foodservice Business Ad 34

Chapter 4 Becoming a Culinary Professional

Section 4.1 Employability Skills

Mathematics Project—Make Customer Change 37

Section 4.2 Seeking Employment

Culinary Skills Project—Evaluate Job Offers.......... 38

Section 4.3 On the Job

English Language Arts Project—List Job Duties.... 39

Study Skills—Getting the Most out of Your Reading 40

Certification Test Practice—Taking Multiple-Choice Tests...................................... 41

Content and Academic Vocabulary..................... 42

Culinary Review—Learn to Network 43

Chapter 5 Customer Service

Section 5.1 Service Basics

English Language Arts Project—Demonstrate Service Skills 46

Section 5.2 Serving Customers

English Language Arts Project—Highlight and Upsell a Menu 47

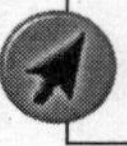

For additional projects and study tools, visit this book's Online Learning Center at glencoe.com.

Contents

Study Skills—Using Critical Thinking Skills............ 48

Certification Test Practice—Taking Fill-In-the-Blank Tests 49

Content and Academic Vocabulary............ 50

Culinary Review—Practice Service Skills............ 51

Chapter 6 The Dining Experience

Section 6.1 Dining Today

Social Studies Project—Determine Service Styles............ 54

Section 6.2 The Dining Room Environment

Culinary Skills Project—Set a Cover............ 55

Study Skills—Preparing for Class............ 56

Certification Test Practice—Taking Short-Answer Tests............ 57

Content and Academic Vocabulary............ 58

Culinary Review—Set a Table............ 59

Unit 2 The Foodservice Industry

Competitive Events Practice—Serving Russian Style............ 62

Chapter 7 Foodservice Management

Section 7.1 Management Basics

Culinary Skills Project—Manage Foodservice Staff............ 64

Section 7.2 Managing People and Facilities

Mathematics Project—Set Production Schedules............ 65

Section 7.3 Foodservice Marketing

English Language Arts Project—Assess a Competitor............ 66

Study Skills—Taking Notes During Class............ 67

Certification Test Practice—Taking Essay Tests............ 68

Content and Academic Vocabulary............ 69

Culinary Review—Set a Floor Plan and Schedule............ 70

Chapter 8 Standards, Regulations, and Laws

Section 8.1 Foodservice Standards and Regulations

Social Studies Project—Name Regulatory Agencies............ 73

Section 8.2 Employment Laws

Social Studies Project—The Americans With Disabilities Act............ 74

Study Skills—Revising Notes............ 75

Certification Test Practice—Understanding Essay Test Words............ 76

Content and Academic Vocabulary............ 77

Culinary Review—Use the Food Code............ 78

Unit 3 Quality Foodservice Practices

Competitive Events Practice—Team Management............ 81

Chapter 9 Equipment and Technology

Section 9.1 The Commercial Kitchen

English Language Arts Project—Organize Kitchen Workflow............ 83

Section 9.2 Receiving and Storage Equipment

Science Project—Clean Refrigerator Shelves............ 84

Section 9.3 Preparation and Cooking Equipment

Mathematics Project—Common Cooking Equipment............ 85

Section 9.4 Holding and Service Equipment

Culinary Skills Project—Identify Holding Equipment............ 86

Study Skills—Studying Your Textbook............ 87

Certification Test Practice—Studying for Tests............ 88

Content and Academic Vocabulary............ 89

Culinary Review—Create a Maintenance Sheet............ 90

Chapter 10 Knives and Smallwares

Section 10.1 Knives

Culinary Skills Project—Identify Knife Construction............ 93

Contents

Section 10.2 Smallwares

Science Project—Choose Measuring Tools 94

Study Skills—Monitoring Comprehension 95

Certification Test Practice—Anticipating Test Questions 96

Content and Academic Vocabulary 97

Culinary Review—Choose Knives and Smallwares 98

Chapter 11 Culinary Nutrition

Section 11.1 Nutrition Basics

Science Project—Choose Nutritious Menu Options 101

Section 11.2 Meal Planning Guidelines

Culinary Skills Project—Read Food Labels 102

Section 11.3 Keep Food Nutritious

Culinary Skills Project—Make Nutritious Choices 103

Study Skills—Staying Healthy 104

Certification Test Practice—Relieving Test Stress 105

Content and Academic Vocabulary 106

Culinary Review—Evaluate Food Choices 107

Chapter 12 Creating Menus

Section 12.1 The Menu

English Language Arts Project—List Factors that Influence a Menu 110

Section 12.2 Menu Planning and Design

English Language Arts Project—Write Menu Descriptions 111

Section 12.3 Pricing Menu Items

Mathematics Project—Compare Pricing Methods 112

Study Skills—Balancing School and Social Life ... 113

Certification Test Practice—Practicing Time Management 114

Content and Academic Vocabulary 115

Culinary Review—Research Menu Types 116

Chapter 13 Using Standardized Recipes

Section 13.1 Standardized Recipe Basics

Culinary Skills Project—Identify Parts of a Recipe 119

Section 13.2 Recipe Measurement and Conversion

Mathematics Project—Convert Equivalents 120

Study Skills—Managing Distractions 121

Certification Test Practice—Eliminating Test Jitters 122

Content and Academic Vocabulary 123

Culinary Review—Use Commercial Scales 124

Chapter 14 Cost Control Techniques

Section 14.1 Calculating Food Costs

Mathematics Project—Choose Scoops and Ladles 127

Section 14.2 Managing Food Cost Factors

Social Studies Project—Assess Regional, National, and Global Factors 128

Study Skills—Using Contextual Definitions 129

Certification Test Practice—Organizing Study Groups 130

Content and Academic Vocabulary 131

Culinary Review—Calculate Food Costs 132

Unit 4 The Professional Kitchen

Competitive Events Practice—Make a Nutritious Dip 135

Chapter 15 Cooking Techniques

Section 15.1 How Cooking Alters Food

Science Project—List Changes to Food 137

Section 15.2 Dry Cooking Techniques

Science Project—Check Baking Progress 138

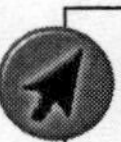

For additional projects and study tools, visit this book's Online Learning Center at glencoe.com.

Contents

Section 15.3 Moist Cooking Techniques

Culinary Skills Project—Make Tomato Concassé.......... 139

Study Skills—Determining Your Learning Style.......... 140

Certification Test Practice—Reviewing After a Test.......... 141

Content and Academic Vocabulary.......... 142

Culinary Review—Evaluate Food Browning.......... 143

Chapter 16 Seasonings and Flavorings

Section 16.1 Enhancing Food

Culinary Skills Project—Determine When to Season.......... 146

Section 16.2 Herbs and Spices

Culinary Skills Project—Identify Herbs and Spices.......... 147

Section 16.3 Condiments, Nuts, and Seeds

Mathematics Project—Compare Charts.......... 148

Section 16.4 Sensory Perception

English Language Arts Project—Evaluate Sensory Appeal.......... 149

Study Skills—Using Note Cards.......... 150

Certification Test Practice—Evaluating Test Results.......... 151

Content and Academic Vocabulary.......... 152

Culinary Review—Taste-Test Seasonings.......... 153

Chapter 17 Breakfast Cookery

Section 17.1 Meat and Egg Preparation

Culinary Skills Project—List Breakfast Food Cooking Techniques.......... 156

Section 17.2 Breakfast Breads and Cereals

Social Studies Project—Research the Pancake.......... 157

Study Skills—Studying in a Group.......... 158

Certification Test Practice—Jogging Your Memory.......... 159

Content and Academic Vocabulary.......... 160

Culinary Review—Produce Breakfast Orders.......... 161

Chapter 18 Garde Manger Basics

Section 18.1 What Is Garde Manger?

Culinary Skills Project—Create a Flower Garnish.......... 164

Section 18.2 Salads and Salad Dressings

Mathematics Project—Cost Food Waste for a Fruit Salad.......... 165

Section 18.3 Cheese

English Language Arts Project—Describe Cheese Use in Recipes.......... 166

Section 18.4 Cold Platters

Culinary Skills Project—Diagram a Fruit Platter.......... 167

Study Skills—Setting Goals.......... 168

Certification Test Practice—Scanning for Information.......... 169

Content and Academic Vocabulary.......... 170

Culinary Review—Build a Salad.......... 171

Chapter 19 Sandwiches and Appetizers

Section 19.1 Sandwich-Making Basics

Culinary Skills Project—Create Nutritious Sandwiches.......... 174

Section 19.2 Sandwiches

Mathematics Project—Cost Tuna Salad Ingredients.......... 175

Section 19.3 Hot Appetizers

Culinary Skills Project—Describe Appetizer Service Types.......... 176

Study Skills—Paraphrasing.......... 177

Certification Test Practice—Improving Your Attitude.......... 178

Content and Academic Vocabulary.......... 179

Culinary Review—Organize Sandwich Making.......... 180

Chapter 20 Stocks, Sauces, and Soups

Section 20.1 Stocks

Culinary Skills Project—Compare Stocks.......... 183

Section 20.2 Sauces

Science Project—Compare a Roux and a Reduction.......... 184

Section 20.3 Soups

Mathematics Project—Calculate Soup Portions... 185

Study Skills—Giving Examples ... 186

Certification Test Practice—Motivating Yourself ... 187

Content and Academic Vocabulary... 188

Culinary Review—Create a Mother Sauce... 189

Chapter 21 Fish and Shellfish

Section 21.1 Fish Basics

Social Studies Project—Research a Fish Dish... 192

Section 21.2 Shellfish Basics

Culinary Skills Project—Select Fish and Shellfish ... 193

Section 21.3 Cooking Fish and Shellfish

Mathematics Project—Cost Seafood... 194

Study Skills—Interacting in Class ... 195

Certification Test Practice—Using the Four Rs... 196

Content and Academic Vocabulary... 197

Culinary Review—Create Shrimp Dishes... 198

Chapter 22 Poultry Cookery

Section 22.1 Poultry Basics

Science Project—Identify Poultry Characteristics ... 201

Section 22.2 Cooking Poultry

Culinary Skills Project—Compare Poultry Textures... 202

Study Skills—Evaluating Web Sites ... 203

Certification Test Practice—Taking Online Tests... 204

Content and Academic Vocabulary... 205

Culinary Review—Create a Simmered Poultry Dish ... 206

Chapter 23 Meat Cookery

Section 23.1 Meat Basics

Science Project—Evaluate Meat Storage ... 209

Section 23.2 Meat Cuts

Culinary Skills Project—Identify Meat Cooking Methods... 210

Section 23.3 Principles of Cooking Meat

English Language Arts Project—Evaluate a Meat Recipe ... 211

Study Skills—Studying Efficiently ... 212

Certification Test Practice—Improving Reading Comprehension... 213

Content and Academic Vocabulary... 214

Culinary Review—Understand Meat Cuts... 215

Chapter 24 Pasta and Grains

Section 24.1 Pasta

Social Studies Project—Discover Asian Noodles ... 218

Section 24.2 Rice and Other Grains

Science Project—Observe Absorption Rates... 219

Study Skills—Researching Diversity ... 220

Certification Test Practice—Using Self-Reflection... 221

Content and Academic Vocabulary... 222

Culinary Review—Cook and Stuff Pasta... 223

Chapter 25 Fruits, Vegetables, and Legumes

Section 25.1 Fruits

Science Project—Ripen Fruit ... 226

Section 25.2 Vegetables

Culinary Skills Project—Prepare Vegetables... 227

Section 25.3 Legumes

Mathematics Project—Count Beans... 228

Study Skills—Improving Memorization Skills... 229

Certification Test Practice—Using Flashcards... 230

Content and Academic Vocabulary... 231

Culinary Review—Research Potatoes... 232

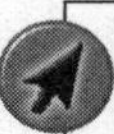

For additional projects and study tools, visit this book's Online Learning Center at glencoe.com.

Contents

Unit 5 Culinary Applications

Competitive Events Practice—Make Chicken Chasseur 235

Chapter 26 Baking Techniques

Section 26.1 Bakeshop Formulas and Equipment

Science Project—Scale Ingredients 237

Section 26.2 Bakeshop Ingredients

Culinary Skills Project—Identify Bakeshop Ingredients 238

Study Skills—Using Mind Maps 239

Certification Test Practice—Taking Open Book Tests 240

Content and Academic Vocabulary 241

Culinary Review—Bake Quick Breads 242

Chapter 27 Yeast Breads and Rolls

Section 27.1 Yeast Dough Basics

English Language Arts Project—Describe Yeast Doughs 245

Section 27.2 Yeast Dough Production

Mathematics Project—Understand Units 246

Study Skills—Preparing for Final Exams 247

Certification Test Practice—Using Old Tests 248

Content and Academic Vocabulary 249

Culinary Review—Form and Evaluate Soft Rolls 250

Chapter 28 Quick Breads

Section 28.1 Making Biscuits

English Language Arts Project—Research Biscuit Recipes 253

Section 28.2 Making Muffins

Mathematics Project—Cost Muffins 254

Study Skills—Improving Concentration 255

Certification Test Practice—Using Test-Taking Strategies 256

Content and Academic Vocabulary 257

Culinary Review—Use Different Blending Methods 258

Chapter 29 Desserts

Section 29.1 Cookies

English Language Arts Project—Summarize a Cookie Recipe 261

Section 29.2 Cakes

Mathematics Project—Calculate Cupcake Combinations 262

Section 29.3 Pies

Culinary Skills Project—Produce Pie Dough 263

Section 29.4 Specialty Desserts

Science Project—Research Gelatin 264

Study Skills—Practicing Good Study Skills 265

Certification Test Practice—Rewarding Yourself ... 266

Content and Academic Vocabulary 267

Culinary Review—Bake Pies 268

Unit 6 Baking and Pastry Applications

Competitive Events Practice—Bake an Angel Food Cake 271

Appendices

Food Safety Rules 273

Kitchen Safety Guidelines 274

Nutritive Value of Foods 275

Name ______________________ Date ____________ Class ________

Chapter 1 Safety and Sanitation Principles

Section 1.1 Safety Basics

Science Project
Describe Sanitation Products

NSES F Develop an understanding of natural and human-induced hazards.

Directions Select one cleaning chemical from each category that is used in your foods lab. Read the bottles and material safety data sheets (MSDS) for these chemicals. Then, complete the chart.

Chemical Name	Equipment on Which to Use	Safety Precautions
Detergent		
Sanitizer		
Degreaser		
Abrasive Cleaner		
Acid Cleaner		

Chapter 1

Name ______________________ Date ____________ Class ____________

Chapter 1

Chapter 1 Safety and Sanitation Principles

Section 1.2 Sanitation Challenges

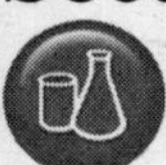

Science Project
List Potential Hazards

NSES F Develop an understanding of personal and community health.

Directions Identify potential biological, chemical, and physical hazards for each area listed in the table below. In the right two columns of the table list the types of hazards and prevention methods for each area. An example has been given.

Foodservice Area	Type of Hazard	Prevention Method
Three-Compartment Sinks	Mold—Biological hazard	Clean sink area; wash and sanitize dishes
Receiving Area		
Refrigerators and Freezers		
Dry Storage Areas		
Cooking Area		
Salad Prep Station		
Baker's Station		
Server Prep Area		

Name ______________________ Date ______________ Class ________

Chapter 1 Safety and Sanitation Principles

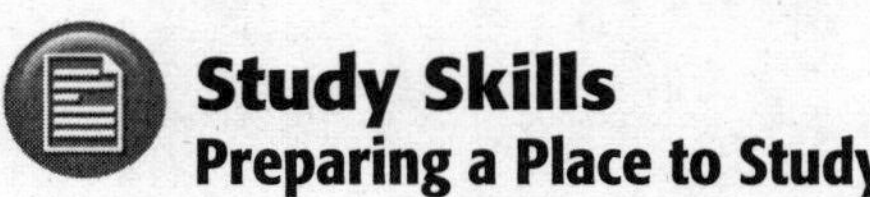

Study Skills
Preparing a Place to Study

Directions Read the tips for preparing a place to study. Answer the questions that follow by making a check mark (✓) for each yes answer. Then, use two or more sentences to describe how well you studied about safety and sanitation.

Tips on Study Spaces
• Designate or create a place where you can be alone. • Ask family members to leave you alone during your study time. • Make sure your study place is quiet, well lit, and a comfortable temperature. • Put all your study materials in your study place. • Add a desk or tabletop to your study place. • Make storage space for your books and materials.

Question	Yes
• Can I be alone in my study place whenever I need to study?	
• Do people respect my study time and leave me alone?	
• Is my study place quiet?	
• Is my study place well lit?	
• Is my study place a comfortable temperature?	
• Are all my study materials in my study place?	
• Is there a desk or tabletop I can use in my study place?	
• Is there storage space for my books and materials in my study place?	

In this chapter, you learned about proper safety and sanitation. How well did your study place help you to prepare for the activities in the chapter? Are there things you might change about your study place to make it more effective?

____

____

____

____

____

____

____

Name ______________________ Date ____________ Class ________

Chapter 1

Chapter 1 Safety and Sanitation Principles

Certification Test Practice
Preparing for Tests

Directions Read the tips for preparing for tests. Then, take the test. Fill in the bubble next to the word that best completes the sentence or answers the question.

Tips for Test Preparation
• Organize the notes you took while reading the text and in class. • Set aside time you will need to study for the test. • Test yourself on the material. • Finish studying the day before the exam. Read it again before you go to bed. • Get a good night's sleep. • On the day of the test, try to relax, be confident, and do your best.

1. __________ helps to keep the workplace safe by writing workplace safety and health standards.
- ○ OSHA
- ○ USDA
- ○ EPA
- ○ FSIS

2. The agency that requires foodservice businesses to trace how they handle and dispose of hazardous waste is __________.
- ○ OSHA
- ○ USDA
- ○ EPA
- ○ FSIS

3. Flammable means __________.
- ○ unable to burn
- ○ on fire
- ○ slow to burn
- ○ quick to burn

4. Fires are classified by __________.
- ○ how big they are
- ○ the type of material that catches fire
- ○ how many fire extinguishers are used
- ○ how hot they are

5. The first thing you should do to treat a serious wound is __________.
- ○ bind the wound tightly
- ○ wash the wound carefully
- ○ call for emergency help
- ○ apply antibiotic ointment

6. You should __________ as soon as possible after an emergency.
- ○ practice an emergency drill
- ○ document any details
- ○ call a friend
- ○ check first aid supplies

Name ______________________ Date ______________ Class ______________

Chapter 1 Safety and Sanitation Principles

Content and Academic Vocabulary
English Language Arts

NCTE 12 Use language to accomplish individual purposes.

Chapter 1

Directions Match each term listed with the correct definition. Write the letter of the term on the line to the left of the definition.

Content Vocabulary		Academic Vocabulary
a. flammable	g. puncture wound	m. routine
b. emergency	h. sanitary	n. document
c. first aid	i. direct contamination	o. result
d. shock	j. cross-contamination	p. transmit
e. laceration	k. toxin	
f. avulsion	l. pathogens	

_______ **1.** A cut or tear in the skin that can be quite deep.

_______ **2.** Clean of dirt, pathogens, and toxins.

_______ **3.** A potentially life-threatening situation that usually occurs suddenly and unexpectedly.

_______ **4.** A serious medical condition in which not enough oxygen reaches tissues.

_______ **5.** Describes any material that is quick to burn.

_______ **6.** The movement of chemicals or microorganisms from one place to another.

_______ **7.** To have an outcome of some kind.

_______ **8.** When the skin is pierced with a pointed object that makes a deep hole.

_______ **9.** A regular set of actions.

_______ **10.** The act of assisting an injured person until professional medical help arrives.

_______ **11.** To write down the details of something that happened.

_______ **12.** An injury in which a portion of the skin is partially or completely torn off.

_______ **13.** To spread.

_______ **14.** When raw foods, or the plants or animals from which they come, are exposed to toxins.

_______ **15.** Disease-causing microorganisms.

_______ **16.** A harmful organism or substance.

Name ______________________ Date ____________ Class ____________

Chapter 1

Chapter 1 Safety and Sanitation Principles

PROJECT Culinary Review
Create a Fire Safety Plan

Scenario Every foodservice workplace should have a fire safety plan to prevent injuries, and even death, from kitchen and dining room fires. In this project, you will create a fire emergency plan for your classroom foods lab. If you do not have a foods lab, you will create a fire emergency plan for your school cafeteria kitchen.

Academic Skills You Will Use	Culinary Skills You Will Use
ENGLISH LANGUAGE ARTS **NCTE 12** Use language to accomplish individual purposes. **NCTE 7** Conduct research and gather, evaluate, and synthesize data to communicate discoveries. **SCIENCE** **NSES F** Develop an understanding of personal and community health.	• Sanitation and safety knowledge • Knowledge of fire safety equipment use • Knowledge of safe kitchen layout

Step 1 Draw an Exit Plan

Directions Carefully examine your classroom foods lab, or school cafeteria kitchen. Draw a diagram of the foods lab or kitchen, marking all large equipment, counters, storage areas, doors, and exits. On your drawing, show where all fire exits are located, mark the location of fire extinguishers, and use a colored pen or pencil to draw the paths people should take to the fire exits.

Name ______________________ Date ______________ Class __________

Chapter 1 Safety and Sanitation Principles

PROJECT **Culinary Review** (continued)
Create a Fire Safety Plan

Step 2 Develop Your Procedure

Directions Read your textbook and answer the questions to develop the information for your fire safety plan.

1. What general actions should someone take if there is a fire? Make a short list.

2. What regular care and maintenance can be performed on areas and equipment in your foods lab to prevent fires? Make a short list.

3. Use the Internet or library to research the stop, drop, and roll technique for putting out a fire on a person. Describe the technique in your own words.

4. Use the Internet or library to research the proper procedure for using a fire extinguisher. Describe the procedure in your own words.

Name ______________________ Date ____________ Class ________

Chapter 1 Safety and Sanitation Principles

PROJECT Culinary Review (continued)
Create a Fire Safety Plan

Step 3 Write Your Plan

Directions Use the information and floor plan you have gathered in Steps 1 and 2 to create a written fire safety plan. Make sure each step is easy to follow. Divide your plan into three sections: Prevention Tips, Safety Equipment, and Escape Plan. Continue on a separate piece of paper, if necessary.

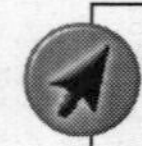

For additional culinary projects and study tools, visit this book's Online Learning Center at glencoe.com.

Name ______________________ Date ______________ Class ____________

Chapter 2 HACCP Applications

Section 2.1 The Safe Foodhandler

Culinary Skills Project

Determining Foodhandler Dress Codes

Directions Read the scenarios about different employees' dress habits. Then, answer the question for each.

1. Julia, a line cook, arrives for her first day at work already dressed for her shift. She is wearing a uniform, an apron, and close-toed shoes. Her hair is loose around her face, and she is wearing long earrings. What would you say to Julia about her outfit?

   ____

   ____

2. Raoul has shown up for his job as a pastry chef with new shoes that are open at the toes. He says they are very comfortable, and will help him to stand all day to do his work. What would you tell him about his new shoes?

   ____

   ____

   ____

   ____

3. Linda has finished cleaning her workspace in the kitchen, and is ready to take out the garbage. What would you advise her about her uniform for this task?

   ____

   ____

   ____

   ____

4. Reagan is dicing onions for a soup, while Joseph is putting garnishes on cold finger sandwiches for a party. Which foodhandler should wear gloves?

   ____

   ____

   ____

   ____

Name ______________________ Date ____________ Class ____________

Chapter 2 HACCP Applications

Section 2.2 The HACCP System

Mathematics Project

Calculate Bacteria Growth

NCTM Number and Operations Compute fluently and make reasonable estimates.

Directions Food items that are between 41°F and 135°F (5°C to 57°C) are in the temperature danger zone because bacteria can multiply rapidly in this temperature range. At 70°F (21°C), bacteria double in number every hour. At 98°F (37°C), bacteria will double every 20 minutes. Complete the chart to calculate the number of bacteria at different times and temperatures for food with minimal initial contamination.

Time	Number of Bacteria at 70°F (21°C)	Number of Bacteria at 98°F (37°C)
12:00 p.m.	1	1
1:00 p.m.		
2:00 p.m.		
3:00 p.m.		
4:00 p.m.		
5:00 p.m.		
6:00 p.m.		

Complete the chart to calculate the number of bacteria at different times and temperatures when starting with contaminated food.

Time	Number of Bacteria at 70°F (21°C)	Number of Bacteria at 98°F (37°C)
12:00 p.m.	1,500	1,500
1:00 p.m.		
2:00 p.m.		
3:00 p.m.		
4:00 p.m.		

Name ______________________ Date ____________ Class ________

Chapter 2 HACCP Applications

Section 2.3 The Flow of Food

Culinary Skills Project
Identify Contamination Hazards

Directions Read the description of each of the following four items. Then, fill in the chart by identifying the type of contamination (direct or cross-contamination), the cause of contamination, and how the contamination could have been prevented.

Item 1 Cartons containing heads of iceberg lettuce on a delivery truck are discolored and are covered with a film.
Item 2 A carton of chicken breasts has been left out on a work table for seven hours.
Item 3 A 10-pound block of cheese in the refrigerator is growing green, fuzzy spots.
Item 4 A cook sneezes on the hamburgers he is preparing.

Type of Contamination	Cause of Contamination	Preventive Measures
Item 1		
Item 2		
Item 3		
Item 4		

Chapter 2

Name ______________________ Date ____________ Class ________

Chapter 2 HACCP Applications

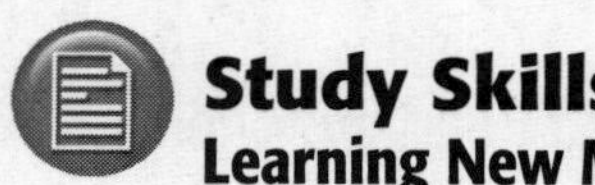

Study Skills
Learning New Material

Directions Read the tips for learning new material. Then, turn each of this chapter's heading into questions relating to food safety guidelines. The first one has been done for you.

Tips to Help Learn New Material
• Preview the material by scanning the chapter objectives, reading guide, headings, figures, photos, and captions. • Think about what you want to learn. • After reading the section, explain the material in your own words.

Chapter 2

Personal Hygiene

1. What is personal hygiene, and how can someone maintain personal hygiene?

Personal Health

2. ______________________________

HACCP Basics

3. ______________________________

System Monitoring

4. ______________________________

Receive and Store Food

5. ______________________________

Preparation and Cooking

6. ______________________________

Disposal Point

7. ______________________________

Name ______________________ Date ____________ Class ________

Chapter 2 HACCP Applications

Certification Test Practice
What to Ask Before a Test

Directions Read the tips for what to ask before a test. Then, complete the sample true or false test. In the table on the right, put a checkmark (✓) under **T** for true or **F** for false.

Questions to Ask Before a Test
Before the day of a test, ask your teacher these questions: • What material will be covered on the test? • What type of questions will appear on the test—multiple choice, true or false, fill in the blank, or essay? • How much time will I have to complete the test? • Will the test be on a computer or in printed form? • Will the test be open book or closed book? • How much will this test count toward my grade for this class?

	T	F
1. Good hygiene is the best defense against cross-contamination.		
2. If you wear gloves or use a hand sanitizer for foodhandling tasks, you do not need to wash your hands.		
3. The HACCP system helps foodservice workers identify foods and procedures that are likely to cause foodborne illness.		
4. The temperature danger zone for foods is 41°F to 135°F (5°C to 57°C).		
5. The flow of food through a foodservice business should be checked by the chef or manager at the end of each day.		
6. Refrigerated foods should be received and stored at a temperature of 41°F (5°C) or below.		
7. Never use a steam table to warm cold food.		

Chapter 2

Name ______________________ Date ____________ Class ________

Chapter 2 HACCP Applications

Content and Academic Vocabulary
English Language Arts

NCTE 12 Use language to accomplish individual purposes.

Directions Write the vocabulary term that best completes each sentence.

Content Vocabulary		Academic Vocabulary
foodhandler	receiving	technique
hygiene	first in, first out	verify
protective clothing	pasteurize	ideal
HACCP	perishable	affect
critical control point	holding	
minimum internal temperature	recycle	

Chapter 2

1. ______________ is the system used to keep food safe on its journey from the kitchen to the table.
2. Accepting deliveries of food and supplies is known as ______________.
3. You should ______________, or check, that the supplies you ordered have not been damaged.
4. To heat a product at high enough temperatures to kill harmful bacteria is to ______________ it.
5. When you take a product at the end of its use and turn it into a raw material to make a different product, you ______________ it.
6. A ______________ is someone who is in direct contact with food.
7. ______________ is worn to help lower the chances of food contamination.
8. When you use the ______________ program, you use food products that are oldest first, before you use newer products.
9. If you put hot foods in the refrigerator, you may ______________ the temperature of the appliance.
10. ______________ products are those than can spoil quickly if not stored properly.
11. The process of keeping foods warm or cold before serving is called ______________.
12. The ______________ is the lowest temperature at which foods can be considered safely cooked.
13. A step in the flow of food where contamination can be prevented or eliminated is known as a ______________.
14. ______________ is using good grooming habits to maintain health.
15. A proper sanitizing ______________ can ensure a safe workplace.
16. Poultry must be kept at the ______________ temperature of 165°F (74°C) for 15 seconds to be considered fully cooked.

Name ______________________ Date ____________ Class ____________

Chapter 2 HACCP Applications

PROJECT Culinary Review
Measure Temperature Correctly

Scenario It is vital to take accurate temperatures of food to help ensure that bacteria does not have a chance to grow and to keep foodborne illness from breaking out. In this project, you will learn how to calibrate a thermometer, review minimum internal temperatures for foods, and keep track of temperatures as a food cooks, holds, and cools.

Academic Skills You Will Use	Culinary Skills You Will Use
SCIENCE **NSES F** Develop an understanding of personal and community health. **MATHEMATICS** **NCTE Measurement** Apply appropriate techniques, tools, and formulas to determine measurements.	• Sanitation and safety knowledge • Thermometer use • Cooking, holding, and cooling

Chapter 2

Step 1 Calibrate a Thermometer

Directions Follow your teacher's directions to form teams. As a team, calibrate a thermometer using these steps. Then, answer the questions.

How to Calibrate a Thermometer
1. Insert the bottom half of an instant-read thermometer stem into a small container of equal parts of ice and cold water. Allow the thermometer to rest. **2.** Read the temperature. The thermometer should read 32°F (0°C). **3.** If the temperature reading in step 2 is not 32°F (0°C), adjust the calibration nut until the thermometer reads 32°F (0°C).

Write a short answer for each question below.

1. Write the definition of calibrate in your own words.

____

____

____

2. Why is it important to calibrate a thermometer?

____

____

____

Name ______________________ Date ______________ Class ______________

Chapter 2 HACCP Applications

PROJECT Culinary Review (continued)
Measure Temperature Correctly

Step 2 Review Minimum Internal Temperatures

Directions In the chart below, list the minimum internal temperatures in degrees Fahrenheit and degrees Celsius, and times for each type of food. Use the information in Chapter 2, and consult the Internet or other research information if needed. If Celsius temperatures are not given, calculate the Celsius temperatures by using the formula (°F – 32) × (5/9) = °C

Food Item	Minimum Safe Internal Temperature/Time
Fish	
Beef, pork, veal, or lamb roasts	
Cooked eggs for immediate service	
Injected meats	
Game meats (commercially dressed game)	
Chopped, ground, flaked, or minced meats	
Fruit or vegetables for hot holding	
Poultry, stuffed meats, and stuffed pastas	
Reheating of foods	
Stuffing	
Microwave cooking of meat, poultry, and fish	

Name ______________________ Date ______________ Class __________

Chapter 2 HACCP Applications

PROJECT Culinary Review (continued)
Measure Temperature Correctly

Step 3 Measure Food Temperature

Directions In teams, prepare a canned cream soup and a canned clear soup according to package directions. Test the soups using your calibrated thermometer for the minimum safe internal temperature for hot holding. Use the first chart to record your results and remedies if the temperature is not safe.

Time and Temperature Checklist			
Food Item	**Safe Temperature Reading**	**Actual Temperature Reading**	**Remedy**
Cream Soup			
Clear Soup			

Use the two-stage cooling method described in Section 2.3 to cool each soup. Take each soup's temperature every 15 minutes, and record your findings in this chart.

Cooling Temperature Chart					
Food Item	**1st Time**	**2nd Time**	**3rd Time**	**4th Time**	**5th Time**
Cream Soup					
Clear Soup					

How can you ensure that each soup maintains a safe temperature during cooling? Write your answer on the lines below.

____

____

For additional culinary projects and study tools, visit this book's Online Learning Center at **glencoe.com**.

Chapter 2

Name ______________________ Date ______________ Class __________

COMPETITIVE EVENTS PRACTICE

Make a Salad

Directions Follow your teacher's instructions to form competition teams of two to four people. Each team will be given a list of basic salad ingredients, and will make a salad using those ingredients. Special attention should be paid to safety and sanitation procedures.

Judging	
In this competition, you will be judged on:	
• How your team handles food safely	• The sanitation procedures you follow
• The appearance and flavor of your salad	• The cleanliness of your workspace

Preparation Phase

1. Write a description of the salad your team chooses to make. Turn in a copy of your description to your teacher.

   ____

   ____

   ____

2. Prepare your workspace for competition. During preparation:
   - Retrieve all necessary equipment and tools
   - Observe all safety and sanitation procedures
   - Keep foods at the proper temperature
   - Use a sanitizing solution to clean your workspace before beginning

   Do not prepare any part of the salad at this time.

Cooking Phase

1. Make your salad, following the description you created. You must make two portions of your salad—one to be tasted, and one for presentation. There should not be a visible difference between the two salads. You will have 30 minutes to make your salads.

2. Bring both salads to the tasting area designated by your teacher when it is completed and ready for judging, or at the end of the time period. Display your salads with the salad description you wrote earlier.

Name ______________ Date ______________ Class ______________

COMPETITIVE EVENTS PRACTICE (continued)

Competitive Events Review

Once the competition has been completed, write a short essay on the experience of competing with other teams. Which parts did you enjoy? Which parts did you not enjoy? What would you have done differently next time?

Name ______________________ Date ____________ Class ________

Chapter 3 Foodservice Career Options

Section 3.1 Careers in Foodservice

English Language Arts Project

Develop a Career Plan

NCTE 7 Conduct research and gather, evaluate, and synthesize data to communicate discoveries.

Directions Complete the steps below to develop a career plan.

1. Using online and print help wanted resources, research the foodservice positions that are available in your community. List six of the jobs that appeal to you the most.

   ____

   ____

   ____

2. Choose one of the jobs, and attach a printed copy of the job description to this activity sheet.

3. Describe your current skills, work experience, and education that would help you get this job.

   ____

   ____

   ____

   ____

4. Describe how you would balance your school activities, social activities, and work if you got this job.

   ____

   ____

   ____

   ____

5. Write out steps you would take to get the training, education, and experience you would need for this job.

   ____

   ____

   ____

   ____

   ____

Chapter 3

Name ______________________ Date ____________ Class ________

Chapter 3 Foodservice Career Options

Section 3.2 Foodservice Trends

Social Studies Project
Track Trends

NCSS V C Individuals, Groups, and Institutions Describe the various forms institutions take, and explain how they develop and change over time.

Directions Investigate trends for foodservice operations in your area. Choose at least three of the operations listed in the box. Identify three trends that impact each operation, and how these trends may affect the operation.

- Quick-service restaurants
- Casual-dining restaurants
- Fine-dining restaurants
- Hotels and resorts
- Banquet facilities
- Government facilities
- On-site catering
- Off-site catering
- Bakeries/pastry shops

Example:

Institutional Dining

A. Increase in quality; better ingredients, more varied recipes

B. Increase in outsourcing; lower costs, increase profits

C. Increase in varied nutritional needs; better variety of ingredients, new cooking techniques

1. Type of Operation:

A. ______________________

B. ______________________

C. ______________________

2. Type of Operation:

A. ______________________

B. ______________________

C. ______________________

3. Type of Operation:

A. ______________________

B. ______________________

C. ______________________

Name ______________________ Date ____________ Class ________

Chapter 3 Foodservice Career Options

Section 3.3 Entrepreneurship

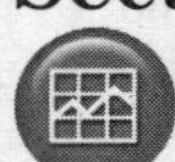

Mathematics Project

Determine Franchise Fees

NCTM Algebra Represent and analyze mathematical situations and structures using algebraic symbols.

Directions Jerry is the owner of a chain restaurant franchise. The table lists Jerry's revenues and expenses for the past three years. Study the table, then answer the questions. (In all equations, assume that f represents the fee, r represents sales revenue, and c represents total costs.)

Revenues and Expenses by Year		
Year 1	**Year 2**	**Year 3**
Sales Revenue $350,000	Sales Revenue $400,000	Sales Revenue $380,000
Food Costs $60,000	Food Costs $70,000	Food Costs $75,000
Labor Costs $180,000	Labor Costs $200,000	Labor Costs $190,000
Overhead Costs $120,000	Overhead Costs $90,000	Overhead Costs...... $85,000

1. If Jerry's contract calls for him to pay the franchise company an annual fee of $10,000 plus 4% of sales revenue, which algebraic equation below correctly represents Jerry's annual fee?

a) $f = 0.04(10{,}000 + r)$ **b)** $f = 10{,}000 + 0.04r$ **c)** $f = 10{,}000 + 4r$

2. How much of a fee did Jerry pay in each year?

Year 1: ____________ Year 2: ____________ Year 3: ____________

3. How much of a profit or loss (after the fee was paid) did Jerry have in each year?

Year 1: ____________ Year 2: ____________ Year 3: ____________

4. If Jerry's contract calls for him to pay the franchise company an annual fee of 8% of profit, which algebraic equation below does not represent Jerry's annual fee?

a) $f = 0.08(r - c)$ **b)** $f = 0.08r - 0.08c$ **c)** $f = 0.08r$

5. Under the contract in question 4, how much of a fee did Jerry pay in each year?

Year 1: ____________ Year 2: ____________ Year 3: ____________

6. How much of a profit or loss (after the fee was paid) did Jerry have in each year?

Year 1: ____________ Year 2: ____________ Year 3: ____________

Name ______________________ Date ____________ Class ________

Chapter 3 Foodservice Career Options

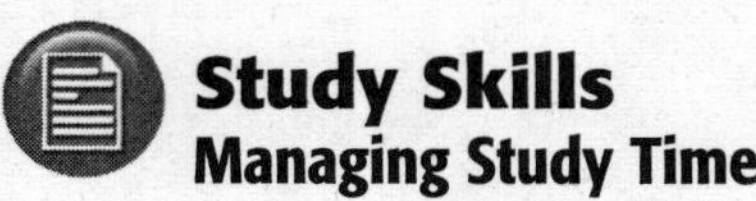

Study Skills
Managing Study Time

Directions Read the tips for managing study time. Then, respond to the prompt to write a paragraph about how good study skills can help you find a career in foodservice.

How to Manage Your Study Time
Do you ever feel overwhelmed by all of the studying you must do? Follow these tips to make your study load more manageable: • Create a schedule for weekly reviews and updates. • Prioritize your assignments. Start with your most difficult task. The other tasks you have to do may seem easier once you have finished the more difficult tasks. • Break big projects into smaller steps. Work on one step at a time. • Reserve some time just before class to review class notes and readings.

Chapter 3 talks about careers, trends, and entrepreneurship opportunities in the foodservice industry. As you decide what career path you want to follow, you assume more responsibility for your choices. This applies to study habits as well. Good study habits can help determine where and how far you may go in your chosen career. Write a paragraph explaining which study habits can help you prepare for a foodservice career.

____

____

____

____

____

____

____

____

____

____

____

____

____

Name ______________________ Date ____________ Class ________

Chapter 3 Foodservice Career Options

Certification Test Practice
Taking True/False Tests

Directions Read the tips for taking true/false tests. Then, take the test. Circle **T** if the statement is true and **F** if the statement is false.

Tips for Taking True/False Tests
• Answer true only when every part of the entire statement is true. If part of the statement is false, the entire statement is false. Watch out for long sentences that include a list or series of statements. Every part of the statement must be true. • Watch out for words that are unqualified, such as always, never, every, or none. These often indicate a false answer. • Statements with words such as usually, sometimes, or often are usually true statements. • Change a sentence written in the negative (no, not, cannot) to a positive by reading the sentence without the negative word. If the statement is true without the negative word, then you know the statement with the negative word is the opposite, or false.

1. Service jobs will not always be available in the foodservice industry. T F

2. Becoming a foodservice manager takes hard work and the right skills. T F

3. The catering director manages the banquet operations of hotels, banquet facilities, hospitals, and universities. T F

4. Hours are very strict at foodservice businesses, so you may have trouble working your classes around your work schedule. T F

5. Foodservice trends may be influenced by society, culture, ethnic diversity, population changes, or the economy. T F

6. Commercial foodservice operations include fast-food chains, fine-dining restaurants, and hospitals. T F

7. There are a wide variety of foodservice jobs available in hotels and resorts because of the wide range of foodservice types available at these locations. T F

8. Three advantages to owning a foodservice or food production business are ownership, job satisfaction, and earning potential. T F

9. Not every business is large enough to need a business plan. T F

10. Free enterprise means that businesses are not subject to any governmental controls. T F

Chapter 3

Name ______________________ Date ____________ Class ________

Chapter 3 Foodservice Career Options

Content and Academic Vocabulary
English Language Arts

NCTE 12 Use language to accomplish individual purposes.

Directions Write the letter of each vocabulary term one the line next to the definition.

Content Vocabulary		Academic Vocabulary
a. kitchen brigade	g. independent restaurant	m. evaluate
b. sous chef	h. chain restaurant	n. analyze
c. certification	i. franchise	o. guidelines
d. entry level	j. business plan	p. accurate
e. trend	k. zoning	
f. profit	l. license	

______ **1.** A job you do not have to have experience or training to do.

______ **2.** A general preference or dislike for something.

______ **3.** To study or examine something to judge its value.

______ **4.** Correct and updated.

______ **5.** A common type of restaurant ownership used by chain restaurants.

______ **6.** A restaurant with two or more locations that sell the same products and operated by the same company.

______ **7.** A written permission to participate in a business activity.

______ **8.** Rules indicating how something should be done.

______ **9.** A group of kitchen staff, each of whom is assigned specific preparation and cooking tasks.

______ **10.** Proof of expertise in a specific topic.

______ **11.** A restaurant with one or more owners that is not a part of a national restaurant business.

______ **12.** A document that describes a new business and a strategy to launch it.

______ **13.** To study all components of something.

______ **14.** A person who supervises and sometimes assists other chefs in the kitchen.

______ **15.** A division of land into sections that can be used for different purposes.

______ **16.** The money a business makes after paying all its expenses.

Name ______________________ Date ____________ Class ________

Chapter 3 Foodservice Career Options

PROJECT Culinary Review
Plan a Foodservice Business Ad

Scenario A business plan can help a foodservice business owner to plan all parts of a business, including advertising. In this project, you will create a fictional restaurant, write out a partial business plan, and create a print ad for your restaurant.

Academic Skills You Will Use	Culinary Skills You Will Use
ENGLISH LANGUAGE ARTS **NCTE 5** Use different writing process elements to communicate effectively. **SOCIAL STUDIES** **NCSS I B Culture** Predict how data and experiences may be interpreted by people from diverse cultural perspectives and frames of reference.	• Foodservice business knowledge • Food trend knowledge • Foodservice advertising knowledge

Chapter 3

Step 1 Create a Fictional Restaurant

Directions Brainstorm the questions below to give you a general idea of the type of foodservice business you will present. Write notes on the lines.

1. What type of food do you want your restaurant to serve?

____

____

____

____

2. How expensive will the dishes on your menu be?

____

____

____

____

3. What types of customers will you serve at your restaurant?

____

____

____

____

Name ______________________ Date ____________ Class ____________

Chapter 3 Foodservice Career Options

PROJECT Culinary Review (continued)
Plan a Foodservice Business Ad

Step 2 Write a Partial Business Plan

Directions Use the information on business plans from Chapter 3 to write a Product and Service Plan and a Market Analysis for a business plan for your fictional restaurant. Use the lines provided, and an extra sheet of paper if you need more room. Be sure to use correct spelling and grammar.

Product and Service Plan Describes the features and benefits of the business's products and services.

____

____

____

____

____

____

____

____

____

Market Analysis Presents your market research and features a customer demographic profile that defines the traits of the company's target market.

____

____

____

____

____

____

____

____

____

____

Chapter 3

Name ______________________ Date ____________ Class ________

Chapter 3 Foodservice Career Options

PROJECT **Culinary Review** (continued)
Plan a Foodservice Business Ad

Step 3 Create Your Ad

Directions Use your Product and Service Plan and Market Analysis as guides to create a print ad for your fictional restaurant. You may use any design elements you wish, but the ad should appeal to your target audience, describe your restaurant accurately, and relate to the information in your business plan.

For additional culinary projects and study tools, visit this book's Online Learning Center at **glencoe.com**.

Chapter 3

Name ______________________ Date ____________ Class ________

Chapter 4 Becoming a Culinary Professional

Section 4.1 Employability Skills

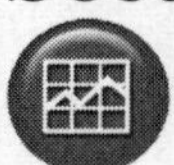

Mathematics Project

Make Customer Change

NCTM Problem Solving Apply and adapt a variety of appropriate strategies to solve problems.

Directions For each item in the Amount of Sale column, calculate the Total Change to the customer. Break down the change into the least number of coins and bills needed to make customer change. Write the information into the correct spaces on the chart.

Amount of Sale	Amount Tendered	Total Change	Penny $0.01	Nickel $0.05	Dime $0.10	Quarter $0.25	Dollar $1.00	Five Dollar $5.00	Ten Dollar $10.00
$7.52	$10.00								
$12.15	$15.00								
$20.52	$21.02								
$18.76	$20.00								
$4.17	$10.00								
$15.38	$20.00								
$32.14	$35.00								
$27.45	$28.00								
$14.01	$20.01								
$37.29	$40.00								
$8.37	$20.00								
$20.28	$30.03								
$15.25	$20.25								
$42.55	$50.00								
$13.11	$20.00								

Name ______________________ Date ____________ Class ________

Chapter 4 Becoming a Culinary Professional

Section 4.2 Seeking Employment

Culinary Skills Project
Evaluate Job Offers

Directions Read each scenario. Evaluate each job offer presented. Then, decide which job offer should be accepted and why.

1. Marianne is a high school career and technical education student. She wants to be a chef someday. Marianne applied for several part-time jobs in foodservice to gain practical experience. She has received two job offers:

Job A Fry station cook	**Job B** Hostess in a hotel dining room

Which should she choose? Explain why. ______________________

____

____

2. Ricardo is 27 years old. He has held a variety of positions in foodservice, and prefers to work in the kitchen. He has received the following job offers:

Job A An entry-level kitchen worker at a fine-dining seafood restaurant averaging 40 hours per week	**Job B** Line cook at a coffeehouse that is open only from 4:00 a.m. to noon

Which should he choose? Explain why. ______________________

____

____

3. Sabrina has eight years of professional pastry chef experience. She is established in the community and is actively involved with local charities. She is seeking more responsibility, but she does not want to relocate. She has received the following job offers:

Job A Assistant pastry chef at a local specialty establishment; her responsibilities will increase, but so will the hours she works	**Job B** Head pastry chef at a hotel restaurant located 30 miles away; her responsibilities will increase, but her hours will not

Which should she choose? Explain why. ______________________

____

____

Chapter 4

Name ______________________ Date ____________ Class ________

Chapter 4 Becoming a Culinary Professional

Section 4.3 On the Job

NCTE 1 Read texts to acquire new information.

English Language Arts Project

List Job Duties

Directions As you read Chapter 4, think about the different on-the-job duties of professional foodservice workers. On the lines, write what you think the everyday duties of each position might include.

Line Cook ____

Restaurant Manager ____

Catering Director ____

Sous Chef ____

Name ______________________ Date ______________ Class __________

Chapter 4 Becoming a Culinary Professional

Study Skills
Get the Most Out of Your Reading

Directions Read the tips for getting the most out of your reading. Then, complete the items listed. In step A, turn the selected heading from Chapter 4 into a question. In step B, write a paragraph in your own words to answer the question, showing that you understand your reading. The first one is started for you.

How to Get the Most Out of Your Reading
• Identify a section of the book that you will read during your study time. • As you read, cover each paragraph that you do not understand with a sticky note. • When you have read through the section, go back and reread all the paragraphs covered with sticky notes. • If you understand the paragraph, remove the sticky note. • Pause to look up definitions of words you do not understand. • Read aloud to clarify concepts that seem confusing when read silently. • If you still have trouble comprehending a paragraph, write your questions on the sticky note and prepare to ask your teacher when you are in class.

1. **a) Work Ethic** What constitutes a good work ethic?

   b) Foodservice employees should maintain a good work ethic because ______________________

   ____

2. **a) Rights and Responsibilities** ______________________

   b) ______________________

   ____

Chapter 4

Chapter 4 Becoming a Culinary Professional

Certification Test Practice
Taking Multiple-Choice Tests

Directions Read the tips for taking multiple-choice tests. Then, take the test. Circle the letter of the answer to each question.

Tips for Multiple-Choice Tests
• Multiple choice questions may present you with answers that seem partially true. The correct answer is the one that is completely true. • Read all answers carefully. Some may seem identical, but a different word can make the difference between right and wrong. • Read all questions carefully. Easy-to-miss terms like is not or are not change the meaning of the question. • If you know for certain that three answers are correct, choose all of the above.

1. Basic skills that employers expect an employee to have include:
a. calculating
b. communicating
c. thinking
d. all of the above

2. Which of these is not a key step of active listening?
a. Think about the purpose of the message.
b. Ask the speaker questions to clarify meaning.
c. Do not watch the speaker's actions.
d. Listen for the end of the message.

3. Friends and classmates can make good networking sources because:
a. They will be doing research on foodservice jobs.
b. They can vouch for your work habits.
c. They know you from classes.
d. They like the same activities as you do.

4. To whom would a job portfolio be given?
a. your school counselor
b. a potential employer
c. the USDA
d. your networking contacts

5. How can you advance in a foodservice job?
a. through a job promotion
b. by getting more responsibilities
c. by getting a better job
d. all of the above

Name ______________________ Date ______________ Class ______________

Chapter 4 Becoming a Culinary Professional

Content and Academic Vocabulary
English Language Arts

NCTE 12 Use language to accomplish individual purposes.

Directions Fill in the right column of the chart with the best vocabulary term from the list. Then, write a sentence in the left column using the word. The first one is completed for you.

Content Vocabulary		Academic Vocabulary
active listening	evaluation	suitable
work ethic	discrimination	field
resource	benefits	

A raw material with which you do your work **1.** Crystal knew her best resource was her ability to work with people.	resource
To have the right qualifications **2.**	
The skill of paying attention and interacting with a speaker **3.**	
Services or payments provided by an employer in addition to wages **4.**	
A personal commitment to doing one's very best as part of a team **5.**	
A written report of how well an employee has performed job duties **6.**	
Line of work **7.**	
Unfair treatment based on age, gender, race, ethnicity, religion, physical appearance, disability, or other factors **8.**	

Chapter 4

Name ______________________ Date ______________ Class ______________

Chapter 4 Becoming a Culinary Professional

PROJECT

Culinary Review
Learn to Network

Scenario Networking involves using personal contacts to find a job. Anyone you know is a personal contact, including friends, family, teachers, students, neighbors, and student or professional organizations. In this project, you will create a networking contact list, statements about yourself and your job search, and network with others.

Academic Skills You Will Use	Culinary Skills You Will Use
ENGLISH LANGUAGE ARTS **NCTE 4** Use written language to communicate effectively. **SOCIAL STUDIES** **NCSS IV H Individual Development and Identity** Work independently and cooperatively within groups and institutions to accomplish goals.	• Foodservice job knowledge • Networking skills

Step 1 Create a Networking List

Directions Consider everyone you know and try to fill in as many names as possible on the chart below. Remember that each person you know also knows people who might help in your job search. Consider any student or professional organizations to which you belong.

Friends and Family	Teachers and Other Students	Neighbors	Former Employers	Student or Professional Organizations

Chapter 4

Name ______________________ Date ____________ Class ______

Chapter 4 Becoming a Culinary Professional

PROJECT Culinary Review (continued)
Learn to Network

Step 2 Express Your Career Goals

Directions Answer the questions to create focused statements about yourself and your career goals.

1. Write a 30- to 40-word statement that tells others who you are. You could include school, family, and hobby information, if it helps you describe yourself in a professional manner. For example, "I'm a junior in high school, I'm outgoing, and I like to be active in the community."

____

____

____

____

____

2. Write a 30- to 40-word statement that outlines your career goals. For example, "I would like to work part time in a foodservice facility until I graduate from culinary school. I hope to become a chef someday."

____

____

____

____

____

3. Write a 30- to 40-word statement that explains what you can offer a foodservice employer. For example, "I am an eager learner and a very patient person. I also have experience working as part of the service staff at a local family-style restaurant."

____

____

____

____

____

____

Chapter 4

Name ____________________ Date ____________ Class ____________

Chapter 4 Becoming a Culinary Professional

PROJECT Culinary Review (continued)
Learn to Network

Step 3 Network with Others

Directions Call or visit five people on your contact list from Step 1. Use your prepared statements from Step 2 to tell them about your foodservice job search. Note their responses on the lines.

Contact 1 ____

____

____

____

Contact 2 ____

____

____

____

Contact 3 ____

____

____

____

Contact 4 ____

____

____

____

Contact 5 ____

____

____

____

For additional culinary projects and study tools, visit this book's Online Learning Center at glencoe.com.

Chapter 4

Name ______________________ Date ____________ Class __________

Chapter 5 Customer Service

Section 5.1 Service Basics

English Language Arts Project
Demonstrate Service Skills

NCTE 1 Read texts to acquire new information.

Directions Read Section 5.1 to learn the service skills needed by foodservice employees who will interact with customers. Then, fill in the chart, listing the service skill, and writing an example of how a foodservice employee might demonstrate that skill. The first one is done for you.

Service Skill	Example
Positive Attitude	A customer has just yelled at Samara because his order was not correct, but Samara keeps her positive attitude by serving other customers without being visibly upset.

Name ______________________ Date ______________ Class ________

Chapter 5 Customer Service

Section 5.2 Serving Customers

English Language Arts Project
Highlight and Upsell a Menu

NCTE 5 Use different writing process elements to communicate effectively.

Directions Read the menu. Then, practice your highlighting and upselling skills by writing a dialogue for a server to highlight and upsell items from the menu.

LUNCHEON MENU

Entrées:

- Baked Chicken Breast Served with Roasted Potatoes and Fresh Green Beans
- Pasta Stuffed with Ricotta Cheese, Covered in a Fresh Tomato Sauce, Served with a Green Salad

Beverages:

- Bottled Mineral Water
- Coffee
- Water

1. **Highlighting** Highlight one of the entrées to entice a customer into ordering it.

____

____

____

____

____

____

2. **Upselling** A customer orders a glass of water. Upsell the water by convincing the customer to purchase bottled mineral water.

____

____

____

____

____

____

____

Chapter 5

Name ______________________ Date ____________ Class ________

Chapter 5 Customer Service

Study Skills
Using Critical Thinking Skills

Directions Read the tips for critical thinking. Then, use critical thinking skills to answer the question.

Improve Your Critical Thinking Skills
Thinking critically is important when taking in new material and information. Practice these tips for improving your critical thinking skills: • Be objective and honest when thinking about and reacting to what you are listening to or reading. • Ask questions and make comments when encountering information. Imagine you are having a conversation with the author when you read. Write down your questions and comments. • Think matters through completely and consider all the information you have before taking a stance or making a decision. • Look for evidence with which to support your beliefs and decisions. • Refrain from being manipulated by what you hear or read. Be aware of biases, subjectivity, and omissions in the author's or speaker's communication.

Critical Thinking Question

Customer service skills are usually one of the first things foodservice employers look for in potential employees. Why do you think customer service skills are so valuable to foodservice businesses? Use your critical thinking skills, and explain your answer in three or four sentences.

Name ____________________ Date __________ Class ________

Chapter 5 Customer Service

Certification Test Practice

Taking Fill-In-the-Blank Tests

Directions Read the tips for taking fill-in-the-blank tests. Then, take the sample test. Use words from the word list to fill in the blanks to complete the sentences.

Tips for Taking Fill-In-the-Blank Tests
• Carefully read the statement and all the word choices before answering each statement. Think about what each word means. • Fill in the statements you are sure about with the best word choice. • The best choice is the one that causes the statement to be factual and reflect what you have learned in your reading. • Cross off words as you use them to avoid using them again. • Once you have eliminated the words you are sure of, review the words you are less sure of and reread each statement. Fill in the blank with the best choice.

positive attitude	upselling	service team
highlighting	position number	demitasse
abbreviations	ingredients	

1. The host, server, busser, and cashier are all part of a restaurant's __________.

2. A server must know the __________ and preparation methods of all beverage and food items.

3. It is critical to have a __________ at all times when interacting with customers.

4. An espresso drink is usually served in a __________ cup.

5. Servers can use __________ to promote specials or regular menu items.

6. Suggesting a larger size of something a customer has ordered is an example of __________.

7. You must learn to use __________, or shortened words that the kitchen staff understands.

8. When you use an order pad, write down the customer's __________ and table number next to each order.

Chapter 5

Name ____________________ Date __________ Class __________

Chapter 5 Customer Service

Content and Academic Vocabulary
English Language Arts

NCTE 12 Use language to accomplish individual purposes.

Directions Use each vocabulary term to write a sentence that shows that you understand the term's meaning. The first one is completed for you.

1. **host** Jeff loved greeting new customers as the **host** of the new organic foods restaurant.
2. **server** ____________________
3. **busser** ____________________
4. **cashier** ____________________
5. **client base** ____________________
6. **uniform** ____________________
7. **cover** ____________________
8. **highlighting** ____________________
9. **upselling** ____________________
10. **hand service** ____________________
11. **tray service** ____________________
12. **preset** ____________________
13. **anticipate** ____________________

Chapter 5

Name ______________________ Date ____________ Class ________

Chapter 5 Customer Service

PROJECT

Culinary Review
Practice Service Skills

Scenario A server should understand how to perform tray service, hand service, and beverage service skills, but these skills take practice to perform correctly. In this project, you will gain a better understanding of service skills, practice those skills, and then perform them for your instructor.

Academic Skills You Will Use	Culinary Skills You Will Use
ENGLISH LANGUAGE ARTS **NCTE 12** Use language to accomplish individual purposes. **SOCIAL STUDIES** **NCSS IV H Individual Development and Identity** Work independently and cooperatively within groups and institutions to accomplish goals.	• Serving skills • Beverage service knowledge • Customer service skills

Step 1 Identify Service Skills

Directions Use the information found in Chapter 5 to describe these three service skills using your own words.

1. **Tray Service** ______________________________

2. **Hand Service** ______________________________

3. **Beverage Service** ______________________________

Name ____________ Date ________ Class ________

Chapter 5 Customer Service

PROJECT Culinary Review (continued)
Practice Service Skills

Step 2 Practice as a Group

Directions Follow your teacher's instructions to form small groups. Practice each type of service skill, following the directions below and the definitions you wrote in Step 1 as a reference guide. Each group member should have the chance to be the server, while others are the customers.

Tray Service Load a large service tray with dishes and glasses filled with water so that the tray is balanced. Take turns properly lifting and carrying the tray to a table. Place the tray on a tray stand, and serve the dishes.

Hand Service Carry three plates on your right arm and a fourth in the left hand to a table. Serve the plates to customers at the table.

Beverage Service Take beverage orders for coffee, hot tea, and iced tea. Fill the proper cups with water, and practice serving the correct beverages to the correct customers.

Once each group member has practiced serving, write your answers to these questions:

1. Which service skill did you find easiest to perform, and why?

2. Which service skill did you find the most challenging to perform, and why?

3. Which skills will you need to practice more, and how can you improve?

Chapter 5

Name ______________________ Date ______________ Class __________

Chapter 5 Customer Service

PROJECT Culinary Review (continued)
Practice Service Skills

Step 3 Demonstrate Your Skills

Directions Perform the service skills you practiced in tray service, hand service, and beverage service for your instructor. Once you have finished demonstrating your skills, answer the essay question.

Why do you think it is important for servers to practice different types of service skills? How does it help restaurants to have well-trained servers?

____

____

____

____

____

____

____

____

____

____

____

____

____

____

____

____

____

____

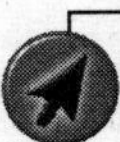

For additional culinary projects and study tools, visit this book's Online Learning Center at glencoe.com.

Name ______________________ Date ______________ Class ______________

Chapter 6 The Dining Experience

Section 6.1 Dining Today

Social Studies Project
Determine Service Styles

NCSS V G Individuals, Groups, and Institutions Analyze the extent to which groups and institutions meet individual needs and promote the common good in contemporary and historical settings.

Directions Read the list of restaurant types. Use the information about serving styles in Section 6.1 of your textbook to determine which serving style or styles would be most appropriate for each type of restaurant. Write your choices on the lines, and explain your choices.

1. **Casual-Dining Restaurant**

   Service Style(s)

   ____

   ____

2. **Fine-Dining Restaurant**

   Service Style(s)

   ____

   ____

   ____

3. **Banquet Hall**

   Service Style(s)

   ____

   ____

4. **Themed Restaurant**

   Service Style(s)

   ____

   ____

5. **Buffet**

   Service Style(s)

   ____

   ____

   ____

Name ______________________ Date ______________ Class ___________

Chapter 6 The Dining Experience

Section 6.2 The Dining Room Environment

Culinary Skills Project

Set a Cover

Directions In the drawing, label the correct placement for the tableware for a dinner. Include all of the items listed.

1. Dinner plate	**7.** Bread-and-butter plate
2. Napkin	**8.** Butter knife
3. Salad fork	**9.** Water glass
4. Dinner fork	**10.** Beverage glass
5. Dinner knife	**11.** Coffee cup and saucer
6. Teaspoon	**12.** Dessert fork and spoon

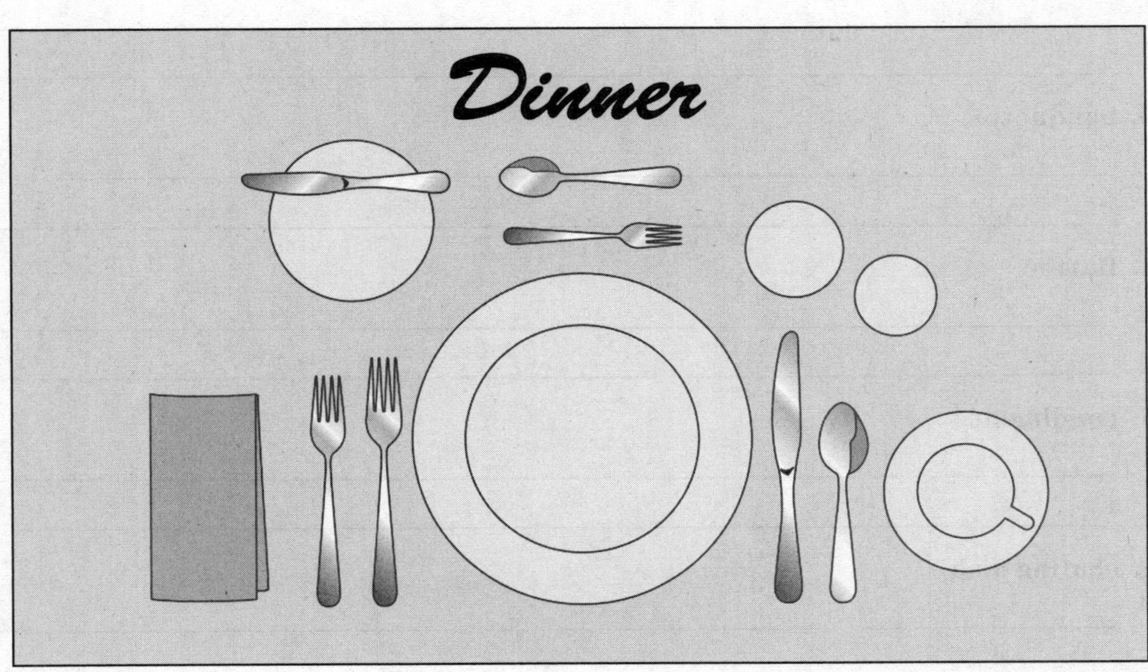

Name ______________________ Date ____________ Class __________

Chapter 6

Chapter 6 The Dining Experience

Study Skills

Preparing for Class

Directions Read the tips for preparing for class. Then, get a head start on your notes for this chapter by writing down some of the key content and academic vocabulary terms in this chapter, looking up their definitions, and writing them.

How to Prepare for Class
• Come to class with your homework completed. • Skim any material you have read to prepare for today. • Review your notes from the previous lecture. • Talk to your teacher about any problems you are having with the material. • Have your notebook and pen or pencil ready for note taking.

1. **trayline service**

____

____

2. **food court**

____

____

3. **banquette**

____

____

4. **flambé**

____

____

5. **condiment**

____

____

6. **chafing dish**

____

____

7. **serviette**

____

____

Name ______________________ Date ______________ Class ________

Chapter 6 The Dining Experience

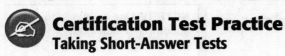

Certification Test Practice

Taking Short-Answer Tests

Chapter 6

Directions Read the tips for taking short-answer tests. Then, take the test. Write a short answer for each question.

Tips for Taking Short-Answer Tests

A teacher's purpose with a short answer test is to see if students know the material well enough to discuss it in their own words. To succeed on a short answer test:

- Prepare by writing about the main ideas you will be tested on in your own words with your book closed.
- When you study, focus on information and concepts, not memorizing exact wording.
- Write your answers legibly in the spaces provided.
- Do not worry about using complete sentences on short answer tests unless your teacher asks you to do so.

1. What are the features of a themed restaurant?

____

____

2. How are catering services provided under contract foodservice?

____

____

3. Explain how to serve beverages and soup in modern American plated service.

____

____

4. What is one advantage of using family service?

____

____

5. To what does the atmosphere of a restaurant refer?

____

____

6. How should coffee cups be preset on a table?

____

____

Name ________________ Date ________ Class ________

Chapter 6 The Dining Experience

Content and Academic Vocabulary
English Language Arts

NCTE 12 Use language to accomplish individual purposes.

Directions Choose the vocabulary term from the list that best completes each sentence. Write the word in the right column of the chart.

Content Vocabulary		Academic Vocabulary
fine-dining restaurant casual-dining restaurant Russian/English service butler service	side work glassware flatware	promote device

Definition	Example	Word
To advertise	The new Korean restaurant gave samples of ribs to passersby to ____________ its menu.	
A restaurant for people who want a less-formal atmosphere and lower prices	The Garber family preferred to eat in a ____________ because of its relaxed atmosphere.	
Duties that service staff members perform before the dining room is open to customers	Lisa and Noel cleaned and refilled the sugar bowls as part of their ____________.	
Dining utensils, such as spoons, forks, and knives	Opal chose a classic pattern of ____________ in stainless steel.	
A style of serving in which the server carries food on a tray to customers, and customers serve themselves	Cornelia Vanderbilt always used ____________ during dinners at her estate.	
A restaurant with excellent food, elegant decor, and superior service	George made reservations at a ____________ to celebrate his friend Ariel's promotion.	
An item that serves a function	A food processor is a time-saving ____________ used by many professional chefs.	
A style of serving in which each food item is served individually in portions from a tray to customers	____________ is often used at banquets where everyone is served the same meal.	
Containers for beverages, either lead crystal or heat-treated	The serving staff made certain the ____________ was clean before pouring the beverages.	

Name ______________________ Date ____________ Class __________

Chapter 6 The Dining Experience

PROJECT

Culinary Review
Set a Table

Scenario Setting a table for customers must be done properly, with all utensils, dishes, and glasses in the right place. In this project, you will determine the items you will need to set a table for six customers, draw a diagram of your place setting, and answer questions about setting the table.

Academic Skills You Will Use	Culinary Skills You Will Use
ENGLISH LANGUAGE ARTS **NCTE 3** Apply strategies to interpret texts. **NCTE 1** Read texts to acquire new information.	• Dining environment knowledge • Service styles • Tool and utensil knowledge

Step 1 Choose Your Meal

Directions Follow your teacher's instructions to form small groups. As a group, imagine that you are the service staff at a restaurant. Decide on a meal that you would like to serve to a table of six customers.

Describe the meal you would like to serve.

____

____

____

Look at the place settings pictured on page 156 in your textbook. Which place setting would best fit the meal you have planned, and why?

____

____

____

Make a list of the items you will need to set a table according to your chosen setting. Remember that there will be six customers at the table.

____

____

____

____

Examine the napkin folds on page 153 of your textbook. Choose one for your table, and practice creating it.

Name ______________________ Date ____________ Class ________

Chapter 6

Chapter 6 The Dining Experience

PROJECT Culinary Review (continued)
Set a Table

Step 2 Plan the Table

Directions Use the space provided to draw a diagram of the table for six, and include the table settings you have chosen. Include any extra items on the table, such as napkins and centerpieces.

Name ______________________ Date ____________ Class ____________

Chapter 6 The Dining Experience

PROJECT Culinary Review (continued)
Set a Table

Step 3 Set the Table

Directions As a team, gather the supplies needed for your table setting and set up your table for six as presented in your diagram. Fold your napkins in one of the styles pictured on page 153 of your textbook. Evaluate your own table, and the tables of each of the groups. Then, answer the questions.

1. How well does each table match the diagram each group drew? What are the differences, if any?

____

____

____

____

2. What were some of the challenges of setting your own table?

____

____

____

____

____

3. For what type of foodservice business would your table setting be appropriate?

____

____

____

____

4. Why do you think a good table setting is important in a restaurant setting?

____

____

____

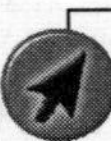

For additional culinary projects and study tools, visit this book's Online Learning Center at glencoe.com.

Name ______________________ Date ____________ Class ________

COMPETITIVE EVENTS PRACTICE

Serve Russian Style

Directions Follow your teacher's instructions to form competition teams of two to four people. Each team will be given directions on how to perform Russian service, and team members will take turns serving a customer using the style. Special attention should be paid to server attitude and correctness of service.

Judging	
In this competition, you will be judged on:	
• How well you are able to serve a customer • Whether you serve from the correct side	• Your attitude as a server • Sanitation and safety principles

Preparation Phase

1. Use your textbook to write a description of how Russian service is performed. Turn in a copy of your description to your teacher.

____

____

____

____

____

2. Prepare your serving tools for competition. During preparation:
   - Retrieve and set up all necessary utensils and dishes in an orderly manner
   - Observe all safety and sanitation procedures
   - Practice using serving spoons
   - Practice using proper manners for customers

Performance Phase

1. Serve a judge using Russian service, following the description you created. Each member of the team should serve an entrée, and then clear the plate from the table. You will have 10 minutes for each team to complete its service.

Name ______________________ Date ______________ Class ______________

COMPETITIVE EVENTS PRACTICE (continued)

Competitive Events Review

Once the competition has been completed, write a short essay on the experience of competing as a service team. How did you coordinate your actions with each other? What did you do to ensure you did not go over the time limit? What would you have done differently next time?

Name ______________________ Date ____________ Class ____________

Chapter 7 Foodservice Management

Section 7.1 Management Basics

Culinary Skills Project
Manage Foodservice Staff

Directions Determine the appropriate management response for each situation below. Write your answers on the lines provided.

Chapter 7

1. **Reassessing Staffing Needs** A line cook calls in sick. What should you do?

2. **Covering the Shift** It is the noon rush, and you are short on staff. You cannot call in anyone else. How do you cover the missing shifts?

3. **Controlling Costs** Flatware is disappearing at the end of the day. How can you address this issue?

4. **Replacing Staff** Three employees have given their two weeks' notice for leaving employment. One other employee no longer shows up for work. What should you do?

Name ______________________ Date ____________ Class ____________

Chapter 7 Foodservice Management

Section 7.2 Managing People and Facilities

NCTM Problem Solving Apply and adapt a variety of appropriate strategies to solve problems.

Mathematics Project
Set Production Schedules

Directions The chart shows a typical production schedule for meal preparation and service. Lunch will be served beginning at 11 a.m. Complete the chart by filling in preparation start times for each menu item. Use the following preparation times to determine the start time for lunch production:

- Country Fried Steak with Gravy—1 hour prep/cook time
- New Potatoes—45 minutes prep/cook time
- Green Beans—30 minutes prep/cook time
- Cloverleaf Rolls—1 hour prep/bake time
- Strawberry Shortcake—2 hours prep/bake time
- Mixed Greens Salad with Ranch Dressing—45 minutes prep time
- Coffee and Iced Tea—15 minutes prep time

Lunch Production Schedule—11:00 A.M. to 2:00 P.M.			
Item	**Portions**	**Work Station**	**Start Time**
Country Fried Steak with Gravy	25	Fry Station	
New Potatoes	25	Hot Station	
Green Beans	25	Hot Station	
Cloverleaf Rolls	50	Bake Station	
Strawberry Shortcake	25	Bake Station	
Mixed Greens Salad with Ranch Dressing	25	Garde Manger Station	
Coffee and Iced Tea	50	Beverage Station and Servers	
Kitchen Clean-Up	N/A	Dishwashing Station	
Floater	N/A	Floater	

Name ____________ Date ________ Class ________

Chapter 7 Foodservice Management

Section 7.3 Foodservice Marketing

English Language Arts Project

Assess a Competitor

NCTE 7 Conduct research and gather, evaluate, and synthesize data to communicate discoveries.

Chapter 7

Directions Choose a local restaurant, and describe its menu offerings and prices. Gather marketing or advertising pieces from the restaurant. Then, answer the questions to analyze the marketing and advertising.

1. Describe the food that the restaurant offers.

2. Describe how the restaurant's marketing and advertising pieces show the restaurant's image.

3. Imagine you are creating a business plan for a new restaurant to compete with this restaurant. How would you position your restaurant differently?

Name ______________________________ Date ____________ Class __________

Chapter 7 Foodservice Management

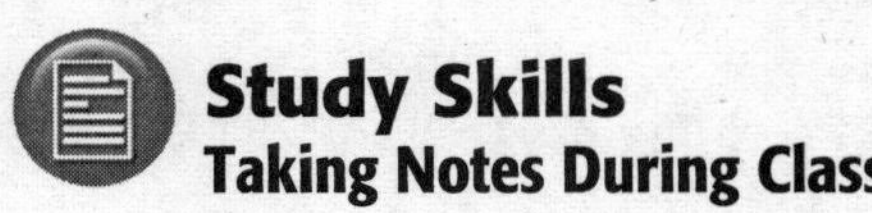

Study Skills
Taking Notes During Class

Directions Read the tips for taking notes during class. Then, use your notes to answer the questions.

How to Take Notes During Class
• Listen actively and concentrate on what your teacher is saying. • Take notes consistently, but do not try to write down every word. • Develop and use a standard method of note taking, such as using an outline format. • Take and keep notes in a large notebook so that they stay organized. • Leave a few blank spaces between one point and another so you can fill in additional information later.

1. Good managers have an ____________ policy with employees, to foster better communication.

2. ____________ is when too many employees are scheduled for a work shift.

3. Employees are given information on the business and its policies during ____________.

4. Good foodservice managers ____________, or give responsibility, to their employees.

5. Effective managers ask ____________ questions during interviews to get more than just a yes or no answer.

6. ______________, including praise for a well-done task, can build employee confidence.

7. Using ______________ can impair an employee's performance on the job.

8. ____________, or the number of times a seat will be occupied during a specific time, must be considered during facility design planning.

9. Many owners develop a ______________ to describe what their business stands for and its main goals.

10. Newspapers, television, radio, and the Internet offer paid ____________ options.

Chapter 7

Name ____________ Date ____________ Class ____________

Chapter 7 Foodservice Management

Certification Test Practice
Taking Essay Tests

Directions Read the tips for taking essay tests. Then, take the essay test.

Tips for Taking Essay Tests
• Essay questions do not necessarily require a lot of writing. Answer the question as precisely as possible. • Give specific information and facts, cite details, and provide examples to support your answer. • In the first paragraph, answer the question directly and state the main points of the essay. You should have two or three points. • In the next two or three paragraphs, explain each of your points with supporting details and examples. • In the last paragraph, summarize the main points and reiterate your answer. • Reread what you have written. Check for spelling punctuation, and clarity.

What are the differences between publicity and advertising?

Name ______________________ Date ____________ Class ________

Chapter 7 Foodservice Management

Content and Academic Vocabulary
English Language Arts

NCTE 12 Use language to accomplish individual purposes.

Directions Write a short essay that uses at least eight of the vocabulary terms in a way that defines what the term means.

Content Vocabulary		Academic Vocabulary
human resources standardized accounting practices food cost percentage income expense inventory	positive reinforcement turnover rate risk management competitor publicity advertising	lapse adhere factor strategy

If I Ran the School Cafeteria

If I ran the school cafeteria, I would definitely make some changes.

Chapter 7

Name ______________________ Date ____________ Class ____________

Chapter 7 Foodservice Management

PROJECT

Culinary Review
Set a Floor Plan and Schedule

Scenario Managing a restaurant requires that you use many different skills. In this project, you will draw a diagram to show the layout of the tables in a dining room, schedule employees in work shifts, and explain your decision-making processes.

Academic Skills You Will Use	Culinary Skills You Will Use
ENGLISH LANGUAGE ARTS **NCTE 7** Conduct research and gather, evaluate, and synthesize data to communicate discoveries. **MATHEMATICS** **NCTM Data Analysis and Probability** Formulate questions that can be addressed with data and collect, organize, and display relevant data to answer them.	• Management skills • Employee scheduling • Dining room design

Chapter 7

Step 1 Draw a Floor Plan

Directions Imagine you manage a small restaurant. In the space below, draw a floor plan of your restaurant dining room. Set the elements listed below within the space. Carefully consider how traffic will flow through the room.

1 bus station
3 smaller tables for two people
2 larger tables for four people
1 kitchen door
1 entrance door

Name ______________________ Date ______________ Class __________

Chapter 7 Foodservice Management

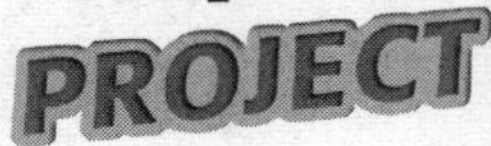

Culinary Review (continued)
Set a Floor Plan and Schedule

Step 2 Create an Employee Work Schedule

Directions Read the information about your restaurant's employees. Then, arrange their work schedules based on that information in the right column in the chart.

Restaurant Employees
• **Dillan** Dillan is a server. He can work a full eight hours, during any shift. • **Jorge** Jorge is a server. He can work six hours, and has requested to work earlier in the day because of an evening commitment. • **Sonia** Sonia is a server and a college student. Because of her class schedule, she can work only four hours. She cannot work first thing in the morning. • **Carol** Carol is a server. She can work a full eight hours, but cannot come in at the beginning of the day. • **Analisa** Analisa is a busser. She can work six hours. • **Eric** Eric is a busser. He can work six hours.

Your restaurant will be open for 12 hours. During that time, no employee may work more than eight hours. You must have three servers working during the lunch rush, which starts at 1 p.m.

Work Schedule 8 A.M. – 8 P.M.	
Employee	**Shift Time**
Dillan	
Jorge	
Sonia	
Carol	
Analisa	
Eric	

Chapter 7

Name _______________ Date _______________ Class _______________

Chapter 7 Foodservice Management

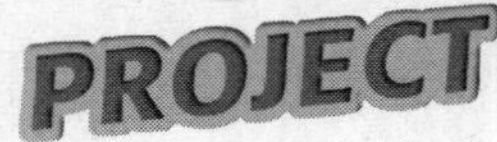

Culinary Review (continued)
Set a Floor Plan and Schedule

Step 3 Analyze Your Management Decisions

Directions Answer the questions based on your experiences from Step 1 and Step 2.

1. What were the biggest challenges in creating a floor plan for a restaurant?

2. What effect do you think traffic flow has on a restaurant's profitability?

3. What were the biggest challenges in scheduling employees for work shifts?

4. Should managers try to accommodate employee shift requests, such as working a specific shift? Why or why not?

5. What types of skills do you think managers must have to perform these tasks on a daily basis?

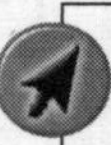

For additional culinary projects and study tools, visit this book's Online Learning Center at glencoe.com.

Name ________________________ Date ____________ Class ________

Chapter 8 Standards, Regulations, and Laws

Section 8.1 Foodservice Standards and Regulations

Social Studies Project
Name Regulatory Agencies

NCSS VIII D Science, Technology, and Society Evaluate various policies that have been proposed as ways of dealing with social changes resulting from new technologies, such as genetically engineered plants and animals.

Directions Look at each example given. Use information from Section 8.1 of your textbook to name the governmental agency responsible for overseeing each example, and name any related foodservice standards or laws.

1. A Prime grading stamp on a package of beef

____

____

2. Percent of daily dietary value on a nutrition label

____

____

3. An irradiation label on a package of fruit

____

____

4. A USDA Food Safety and Inspection Service stamp on eggs, poultry products, or meat products

____

____

5. Health claims on a menu

____

____

6. Foodservice standards for handling food in a professional setting

____

____

7. An employer binder of material safety data sheets for hazardous chemicals

____

____

8. An environmental impact statement for a new restaurant

____

____

Chapter 8

Name ______________________ Date __________ Class __________

Chapter 8 Standards, Regulations, and Laws

Section 8.2 Employment Laws

Social Studies Project

The Americans With Disabilities Act

NCSS VI A Power, Authority, and Governance Examine persistent issues involving the rights, roles, and status of the individual in relation to the general welfare.

Directions Research the Americans With Disabilities Act (ADA) as it relates to foodservice. Then, complete Parts A and B.

PART A Evaluate your foods lab to see if it meets the ADA requirements. How can you improve the flow of the area to make it more accessible to students with disabilities?

____

____

____

PART B Follow your teacher's instructions to choose a partner. Take turns role-playing as a student with a disability and an observer. Choose a disability:

- No left hand or forearm
- Blind
- Walks with a cane
- Deaf

Then, choose a scenario:

- A foodservice handler with a disability needs to prepare side garden salads for lunch.
- A dishwasher with a disability needs to scrape, rinse, rack, and wash dishes in the dishwasher.
- An assistant cook with a disability needs to plate food on the hot food line.

Write your observations of tasks that were easy, moderate, or difficult for the student with the disability. What conclusions can you draw?

____

____

____

____

____

____

____

____

____

____

Chapter 8

Name ______________________ Date ____________ Class ________

Chapter 8 Standards, Regulations, and Laws

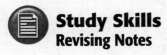

Study Skills
Revising Notes

Directions Read the tips on revising notes. Then, develop a note-taking plan that will work best for you. Write your plan on the lines. Share it with a classmate and exchange ideas.

How to Revise Your Notes
Taking notes in class and while reading the text is an important study skill. You can make your notes more useful by revising them after class or after you have finished reading the text. Follow these tips: • **Recopy your notes.** This helps you organize your notes into main ideas and details. It also gives you the opportunity to make your writing neater and easier to read. Rewriting your notes is more effective than just reading them over. You can also read your notes aloud as you copy them. • **Highlight or color code your notes.** After you copy your notes, develop a system to color code the information. Highlight main ideas in one color and supporting details in another color. Do the same for important vocabulary words: Highlight the words in one color and the definitions in another. • **Use graphic organizers.** Copy your notes into diagrams or visuals that help you organize and remember the information. This can help you see how ideas and information are related. • **Use note cards.** Copy your notes onto separate note cards. Put main ideas on one side and supporting information on the other. Use them like flash cards when you study.

My Note-Taking Plan

___

___

___

___

___

___

___

___

___

___

Chapter 8

Name ______________________ Date __________ Class __________

Chapter 8 Standards, Regulations, and Laws

Certification Test Practice
Understanding Essay Test Words

Directions Read the tips for understanding essay test words. Then, read the prompt and write an essay.

Understanding Essay Test Words
Verbs are key words in essay test questions and directions. Note the difference between the meanings of these verbs, and keep them in mind when completing an essay test or assignment: • To evaluate means to look at the limitations and contributions of an idea. • To justify means to give reasons why an idea was stated. • To relate means to establish connections between concepts or ideas. • To compare means to show how different ideas or concepts are similar. • To contrast means to show how different ideas or concepts are different.

Chapter 8

In an essay, evaluate the effects of FDA regulations on food.

Name ______________________ Date ______________ Class ________

Chapter 8 Standards, Regulations, and Laws

Content and Academic Vocabulary
English Language Arts

NCTE 12 Use language to accomplish individual purposes.

Directions Circle the letter of the phrase that best completes each sentence.

1. A **standard** is
- **a.** a regulation
- **b.** an established model or example used to compare quality
- **c.** a framework or structure
- **d.** a typical group of people or things

2. **Grading** food products involves
- **a.** testing them for safety
- **b.** rating them according to taste
- **c.** applying specific quality standards to them
- **d.** leveling them

3. An **inspection** is
- **a.** a test of a business's practices against standards
- **b.** a cause of anxiety
- **c.** a checkup
- **d.** a strategy

4. If you create an **affirmative action** program, you
- **a.** practice positive reinforcement
- **b.** locate, hire, train, and promote women and minorities
- **c.** promote discrimination
- **d.** promote the rights of men

5. The **Food Code**
- **a.** assigns food products grades
- **b.** is an oath chefs must take
- **c.** gives guidelines for handling food safely
- **d.** is a law regulating food

6. A **disability**
- **a.** is a physical or mental impairment that substantially limits one or more major life activities
- **b.** is a handicap
- **c.** limits a person's ability to seek work or get hired
- **d** limits some employees from receiving the same benefits that other employees receive

7. A **law** is
- **a.** the same as a regulation
- **b.** an established rule
- **c.** a provision
- **d.** the same as a resolution

8. When a foodservice operation is in **violation**, it
- **a.** is following what others are doing
- **b.** is not following a rule
- **c.** is breaking a federal law
- **d.** is in danger of losing profit

Chapter 8

Name ______________________ Date __________ Class ______

Chapter 8 Standards, Regulations, and Laws

PROJECT

Culinary Review
Use the Food Code

Scenario The U.S. Food and Drug Administration's Food Code is used as a guideline for foodservice operations, including management knowledge. In this project, you will read and summarize part of the Food Code, create inspection interview questions, and use those questions to interview another student.

Academic Skills You Will Use	Culinary Skills You Will Use
ENGLISH LANGUAGE ARTS **NCTE 1** Read texts to acquire new information. **NCTE 7** Conduct research and gather, evaluate, and synthesize data to communicate discoveries. **SOCIAL STUDIES** **NCSS V F Individuals, Groups, and Institutions** Evaluate the role of institutions in furthering both continuity and change.	• Sanitation and safety knowledge • Foodservice management skills

Chapter 8

Step 1 Summarize Food Code Information

Directions Follow your teacher's instructions to go online and find the FDA Food Code. Read part 2-102.11 on Management and Personnel: Knowledge: Demonstration. According to the section, what specific types of knowledge must a foodservice manager be able to show?

Name ______________________ Date ____________ Class ________

Chapter 8 Standards, Regulations, and Laws

PROJECT Culinary Review (continued)
Use the Food Code

Step 2 Create Inspection Questions

Directions Use the Food Code knowledge categories and information from Step 1 to create five questions that an FDA inspector might ask a foodservice manager during an inspection. The questions should cover areas discussed in the Food Code section you reviewed. Write out your questions.

Inspection Question #1:

____

____

____

Inspection Question #2:

____

____

____

Inspection Question #3:

____

____

____

Inspection Question #4:

____

____

____

Inspection Question #5:

____

____

____

Chapter 8

Name ______________________ Date ______________ Class ____________

Chapter 8 Standards, Regulations, and Laws

PROJECT Culinary Review (continued)
Use the Food Code

Step 3 Conduct a Management Inspection

Directions Follow your teacher's instructions to form pairs. Take turns asking each other the questions you created in Step 2. First, one student should be the inspector and the other the foodservice manager. Then, switch roles. After you have finished, answer the questions.

1. Which questions were the most difficult for you to answer as a foodservice manager?

____

____

____

____

____

____

2. How might a foodservice manager get more information on these topics?

____

____

____

____

____

____

3. Why do you think it is important for a foodservice manager to be able to answer questions like these during an inspection?

____

____

____

____

____

____

Chapter 8

Name ______________________ Date __________ Class __________

COMPETITIVE EVENTS PRACTICE

Team Management

Directions Follow your teacher's instructions to form competition teams of two people. One team member will manage the other team member as he or she makes a sandwich. The sandwich recipe will be chosen by your teacher. Special attention should be paid to management skills, giving clear directions, and communication between team members.

Judging
In this competition, you will be judged on:
• How effectively the managing team member directs the process • The communication skills between the two team members • The sanitation procedures you follow as you make the sandwich • The cleanliness of your workspace

Preparation Phase

1. As a team, write a work plan of the steps that it will take to make the sandwich. Turn in a copy of your work plan to your teacher.

____

____

____

____

2. Prepare your workspace for competition. During preparation:
   - Retrieve all necessary equipment and tools
   - Observe all safety and sanitation procedures
   - Keep foods at the proper temperature
   - Decide which team member will perform which part
   - Decide how to explain your sandwich-making steps

   Do not prepare any part of the sandwich at this time.

Cooking Phase

1. Make your sandwich, following the work plan you created. The managing team member must accurately describe each step to the sandwich-making team member. He or she should also answer any questions posed by the sandwich-making team member. You will have 10 minutes to make your sandwich.

Name ____________ Date ____________ Class ____________

COMPETITIVE EVENTS PRACTICE (continued)

Competitive Events Review

Once the competition has been completed, answer the questions on the experience of managing another team member, or being managed.

1. If you were the managing team member, what was it like to give direction to someone else?

2. If you were the sandwich-making team member, what was it like to take direction from someone else?

3. What things might you do differently next time?

4. Do you think good communication skills are important between managers and employees? Why or why not?

Name ______________________ Date ______________ Class ________

Chapter 9 Equipment and Technology

Section 9.1 The Commercial Kitchen

NCTE 12 Use language to accomplish individual purposes.

English Language Arts Project
Organize Kitchen Workflow

Directions Walk through your foods lab. If your lab is not set up like a commercial facility, walk through your school's cafeteria kitchen. Suggest changes that might better organize the foods lab or kitchen facility, such as overhead and under-counter storage, adjustments to the cooking line, and any related safety and lighting requirements. Write your suggestions on the lines.

Chapter 9

Name ______________________ Date ______________ Class __________

Chapter 9 Equipment and Technology

Section 9.2 Receiving and Storage Equipment

NCSS A Develop abilities necessary to do scientific inquiry.

Science Project
Clean Refrigerator Shelves

Directions Follow the directions in the box to experiment with cleaning food from refrigerator shelves. Then, answer the questions.

Experiment: Cleaning Refrigerator Shelves

1. Clean three spots on one of your refrigerator shelves.
2. Apply three small spots of tomato sauce.
3. Using standard kitchen cleaning equipment and solutions, clean the spots according to the following schedule:
   - Clean the first spot immediately.
   - Clean the second spot after one day.
   - Clean the third spot after two days.

Once you have completed the experiment, answer these questions:

1. Which spot was the easiest to clean?

____

____

2. Which spot was the most difficult to clean?

____

____

3. Explain why you think your results turned out the way they did.

____

____

____

4. How can you use these results to improve kitchen safety and sanitation?

____

____

____

____

Chapter 9

Name ______________________ Date ____________ Class __________

Chapter 9 Equipment and Technology

Section 9.3 Preparation and Cooking Equipment

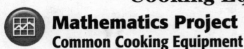

Mathematics Project
Common Cooking Equipment

NCTM Data Analysis and Probability Formulate questions that can be addressed with data and collect, organize, and display relevant data to answer them.

Directions This chart shows the results of a fictional survey of local restaurants that were asked about cooking equipment. Study the chart, and then answer the questions.

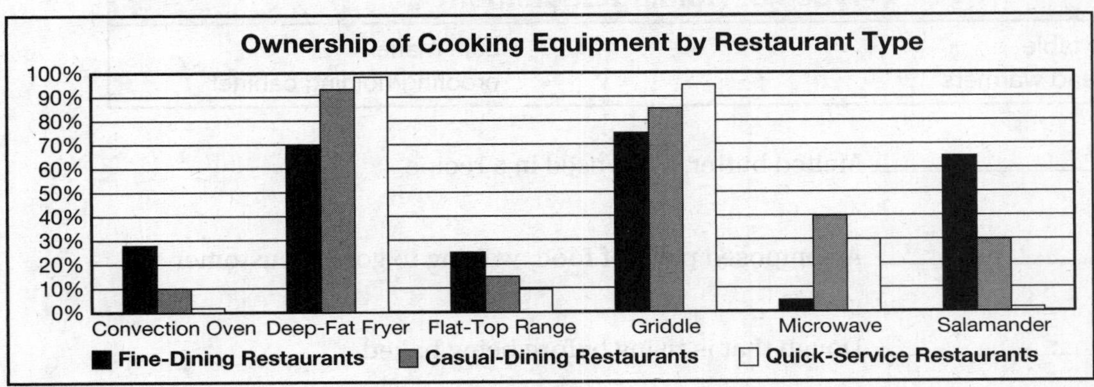

1. Which type of equipment was owned by the most fine-dining restaurants?
   a) salamander b) griddle c) deep-fat fryer d) microwave

2. Which type of equipment was owned by the fewest casual-dining restaurants?
   a) convection oven b) microwave c) salamander d) flat-top range

3. Which type of equipment was owned more frequently by casual-dining restaurants than by other restaurant types?
   a) deep-fat fryer b) microwave c) griddle d) salamander

4. What piece of equipment was owned by more than 70% of all restaurants?
   a) salamander b) deep-fat fryer c) flat-top range d) griddle

5. If 250 quick-service restaurants responded to the survey, which number best represents the total number of those respondents that owned a microwave?
   a) 100 b) 8 c) 75 d) 65

Chapter 9

Name ______________________ Date ____________ Class ____________

Chapter 9 Equipment and Technology

Section 9.4 Holding and Service Equipment

Culinary Skills Project
Identify Holding Equipment

Directions Read the list of the different types of holding equipment. Then, fill in the blanks to show which type of holding equipment would be used for each type of food.

Types of Holding Equipment	
steam table	bain marie
overhead warmers	proofing/holding cabinet

1. ____________ Melted butter, to be used in a recipe
2. ____________ A composed plate of food, waiting to go to a customer
3. ____________ Dough that is rising before being baked
4. ____________ Cooked rice for a buffet
5. ____________ A plate of pancakes, waiting for an order of sausages
6. ____________ Cooked shredded pork for burritos
7. ____________ A crème brulée, needing to be baked
8. ____________ A hotel pan full of vegetables, waiting to go to a steam table
9. ____________ Cashew chicken at a quick-service restaurant
10. ____________ A sheet of freshly baked rolls waiting for a banquet dinner
11. ____________ Chocolate to be used as a liquid garnish for a dessert
12. ____________ A basket of warm rolls waiting to go to a table

Chapter 9

Name ______________________ Date ____________ Class __________

Chapter 9 Equipment and Technology

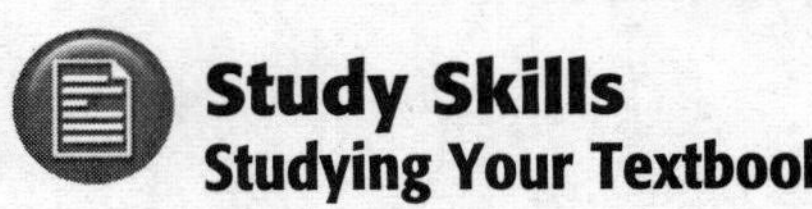

Study Skills
Studying Your Textbook

Directions Read the tips for studying your textbook. Answer the questions by selecting the term or phrase that best completes each sentence. Circle the letter of the correct answer.

Tips for Studying Your Textbook
• After reading a section in your textbook, reread such features as the section introduction and summary. This will help you find the main ideas. • Read section and chapter study questions. Find specific details to answer the questions. • Pay attention to any graphs or tables. Take advantage of the visual aids because they make information visible and easier to understand. • Always read any vocabulary lists at the end of the chapter. Make sure you know the definition of each term. Review the chapter or check the glossary if there are any terms you are unsure of.

1. Mise en place includes all of the following steps except
- **a.** assembling all necessary equipment
- **b.** assembling all necessary tools
- **c.** preparing any food to be used
- **d.** properly cleaning the work station after cooking is completed

2. FIFO stands for
- **a.** food in, food out.
- **b.** first in, first out.
- **c.** first invoice, following order.
- **d.** first in, fifth out.

3. A document that asks a supplier to send food and supplies at a predetermined price is a(n)
- **a.** purchase order.
- **b.** invoice.
- **c.** receiving record.
- **d.** work order.

4. Heating food through direct contact between a hot surface and the food is called
- **a.** convection.
- **b.** conduction.
- **c.** radiation.
- **d.** induction.

5. Holding equipment should hold food at a minimum temperature of
- **a.** 125°F (52°C).
- **b.** 130°F (54°C).
- **c.** 135°F (57°C).
- **d.** 140°F (60°C).

Name ______________________ Date ______________ Class ______________

Chapter 9 Equipment and Technology

Certification Test Practice

Studying for Tests

Directions Use these tips on how to study for tests when studying for an exam. Then, answer the questions.

How to Study for Tests
• Eat something to give you energy to study. Try to avoid excess sugar. An apple does a better job of keeping you focused and awake than caffeine. • Study in a well-lit place that has no distractions, but do not get too comfortable or you may fall asleep. • Keep a positive attitude. It is easier to study when you are relaxed than when you are stressed. • Focus on the main ideas. Skip the details first, but come back to them after you have learned the key points.

1. What are the five different cooking line configurations?

____

____

2. How does having an efficient range of motion help you in the kitchen?

____

____

____

3. What is freezer burn, and how do you prevent it?

____

____

____

4. How is a garbage disposal used?

____

____

5. Where can you use serving equipment?

____

____

Chapter 9

Name ____________________ Date ____________ Class ____________

Chapter 9 Equipment and Technology

Content and Academic Vocabulary

English Language Arts

NCTE 12 Use language to accomplish individual purposes.

Directions Write the correct content or academic vocabulary term on the line next to the definition. The first one is done for you.

Content Vocabulary		Academic Vocabulary
work station	counter scale	efficient
work section	conduction	refer
cooking line	convection	
mise en place	microwave	
purchase order	bain marie	
invoice		

cooking line The arrangement of the kitchen equipment

____________ To reread briefly; to consult a source for information

____________ An invisible wave of energy that causes water molecules to rub against each other and produce heat that cooks food

____________ Heating food by direct contact between a hot surface and the food

____________ A work area that contains the necessary tools and equipment to prepare certain types of food

____________ Assembling all the necessary ingredients, equipment, tools, and serving pieces needed to prepare food, in the order in which they will be used

____________ Productive; well organized

____________ A water bath, used to keep foods warm

____________ Similar work stations grouped into larger work areas

____________ A bill from a supplier for providing goods and services

____________ A document requesting a supplier to ship food or supplies at a predetermined price

____________ Heating food by the circulation of heated molecules of hot liquid or air

____________ A small scale with a platform

Name ______________________ Date ____________ Class ____________

Chapter 9 Equipment and Technology

PROJECT

Culinary Review
Create a Maintenance Sheet

Scenario Keeping equipment clean and in good repair is essential to running a professional kitchen. In this project, you will choose a piece of kitchen equipment, research information on cleaning and maintenance, and then create a maintenance sheet for that piece of equipment.

Academic Skills You Will Use	Culinary Skills You Will Use
ENGLISH LANGUAGE ARTS **NCTE 8** Use information resources to gather information and create and communicate knowledge. **SCIENCE** **NCSS E** Develop understandings about science and technology.	• Sanitation and safety knowledge • Equipment use • Equipment care and maintenance

Step 1 Choose Your Equipment

Directions Look at the equipment pictured in Chapter 9 of your textbook. Choose one piece of equipment, and answer the questions.

1. Which equipment did you choose?

____

2. How does the equipment work?

____

____

____

____

____

3. What foods would you use with the equipment?

____

____

____

____

____

Chapter 9

Name ______________________ Date ____________ Class __________

Chapter 9 Equipment and Technology

PROJECT Culinary Review (continued)
Create a Maintenance Sheet

Step 2 Research Care and Maintenance

Directions Follow your teacher's directions to use the Internet and other sources to research how to properly maintain your chosen equipment. Take notes on daily, weekly, and monthly care recommendations for your equipment. Use this space to organize your notes.

Chapter 9

Name ______________________ Date ______________ Class __________

Chapter 9 Equipment and Technology

PROJECT Culinary Review (continued)
Create a Maintenance Sheet

Step 3 Create a Maintenance Sheet

Directions Use the information you have gathered in Step 2 to create a maintenance sheet for your equipment. List steps to take daily, weekly, and monthly. Use language that could be clearly understood by a new foodservice employee.

Daily Care: ____

____

____

____

____

____

____

Weekly Care: ____

____

____

____

____

____

____

Monthly Care: ____

____

____

____

____

____

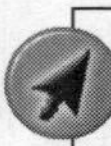
For additional culinary projects and study tools, visit this book's Online Learning Center at **glencoe.com.**

Chapter 9

Name ______________________ Date ____________ Class ________

Chapter 10 Knives and Smallwares

Section 10.1 Knives

Culinary Skills Project

Identify Knife Construction

Directions Label the parts of the knife, as shown in the drawing.

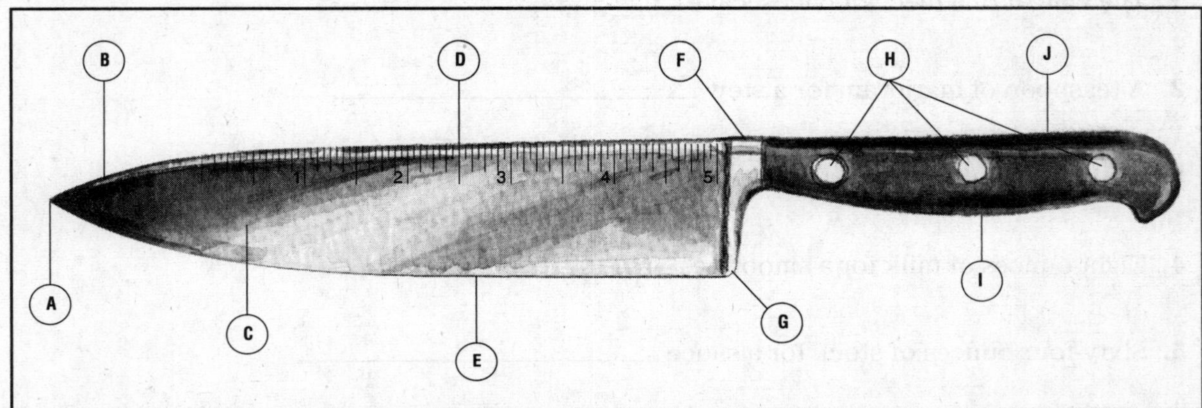

A. ______________

B. ______________

C. ______________

D. ______________

E. ______________

F. ______________

G. ______________

H. ______________

I. ______________

J. ______________

Name ______________________ Date ____________ Class __________

Chapter 10 Knives and Smallwares

Section 10.2 Smallwares

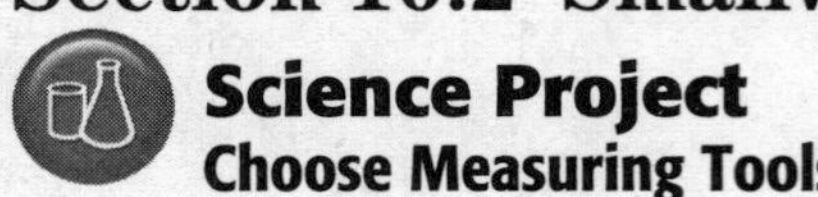

Science Project
Choose Measuring Tools

NCSS 1 Develop an understanding of science unifying concepts and processes: change, constancy, and measurement.

Directions Read the ingredients and foods listed. Use the information in Section 10.2 of your textbook to determine what types of measuring equipment would be needed for each ingredient or food.

1. The weight of a piece of cheesecake ______________________
2. A teaspoon of marjoram for a stew ______________________
3. Gravy for a turkey dinner ______________________
4. Eight ounces of milk for a smoothie ______________________
5. Sixty-four ounces of stock for a sauce ______________________
6. Sixteen ounces of flour for a sheet cake ______________________
7. Three tablespoons of chili powder for chili ______________________
8. Ten ounces of soup ______________________
9. Two quarts of milk for pudding ______________________
10. Fifteen ounces of dough for a quick bread ______________________
11. Three ounces of meatloaf for a single dinner plate ______________________
12. Thirty-six ounces of water for boiling pasta ______________________
13. Two quarts of stock for a risotto recipe ______________________
14. One teaspoon of vanilla extract for a cake ______________________
15. Five ounces of sauce for a pasta dish ______________________

Name ______________________ Date ______________ Class ____________

Chapter 10 Knives and Smallwares

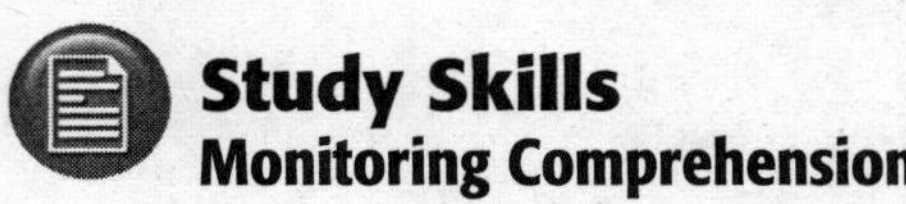

Study Skills
Monitoring Comprehension

Directions Read the tips on monitoring reading comprehension. Then, answer the questions.

How to Monitor Reading Comprehension
While you read your text, it is important to stop occasionally to monitor how well you understand what you are reading. When you stop, ask yourself these questions: • Can I put the main ideas into my own words? • Do I need to look up any words to be sure of their meanings? • Do I understand how the new information relates to the information I have already learned? • Do I need to read any sections over again? • Can I predict what will happen next?

1. In your own words, summarize the main ideas of Chapter 10.

2. What words in Chapter 10 do you not know the meaning of? List them and use a dictionary to write a definition for each one.

3. Why is it important to cut food into uniform pieces?

4. How does heat transfer affect the choice of cookware for a kitchen?

Name ______________________ Date ______________ Class ________

Chapter 10 Knives and Smallwares

Certification Test Practice
Anticipating Test Questions

Directions Read the tips for anticipating test questions. Then, complete the short-answer test. The first one is done for you.

Tips to Anticipate Test Questions
By following these tips, you may be able to accurately predict what your teacher will include on an upcoming test. • Pay close attention to the material that the teacher goes over before the test. • Listen for key points and key words. • Ask your teacher what type of questions you should expect on the test, such as true/false, multiple choice, short answer, or essay. • Ask your teacher what textbook pages you should study for the test. • Watch for clues from your teacher that indicate what may be on the test: o pausing before or after an idea o using repetition to emphasize a point o asking the class questions about the material o writing information on the board o saying, "This will be on the test."

Questions	Short Answers
What is the part of the knife blade that continues into the handle?	the tang
What type of knife is used to trim off the skin from small vegetables?	
Which cut is used to finely slice or shred leafy vegetables or herbs?	
Mincing is used most often on which foods?	
From what materials are the majority of hand tools made?	
What organization tests hand tools for construction, comfort, and safety?	
What tool is used to remove tiny strips from the outer surface of citrus peels?	
What materials are used to make rolling pins?	

Chapter 10

Name ______________________ Date ____________ Class ________

Chapter 10 Knives and Smallwares

Content and Academic Vocabulary
English Language Arts

NCTE 12 Use language to accomplish individual purposes.

Directions Write a description of a visual representation that will help you remember these vocabulary terms. An example is completed for you.

Content Vocabulary		Academic Vocabulary
rondelle	smallwares	uniform
diagonal	weight	withstand
julienne	volume	gauge
batonnet	heat transfer	
trueing		

1. rondelle a circle
2. batonnet ______________________
3. weight ______________________
4. diagonal ______________________
5. gauge ______________________
6. volume ______________________
7. smallwares ______________________
8. truing ______________________
9. heat transfer ______________________
10. uniform ______________________
11. withstand ______________________
12. julienne ______________________

Chapter 10

Name ______________________________ Date ______________ Class __________

Chapter 10 Knives and Smallwares

PROJECT

Culinary Review
Choose Knives and Smallwares

Scenario It is important to choose the correct knives and smallwares for tasks required in a recipe. This will help ensure that the food comes out the same way each time. In this project, you will find a recipe, determine what tasks must be done for that recipe, and then choose the correct knives and smallwares for the tasks.

Academic Skills You Will Use	Culinary Skills You Will Use
ENGLISH LANGUAGE ARTS **NCTE 8** Use information resources to gather information and create and communicate knowledge. **SCIENCE** **NSES 1** Develop an understanding of science unifying concepts and processes: change, constancy, and measurement.	• Reading recipes • Mise en place for recipes • Knives and smallwares knowledge

Step 1 Find a Recipe

Directions Use resources such as the library and the Internet to find a recipe that requires some preparation of the ingredients before cooking. Write out the recipe in the space provided.

Chapter 10

Name ______________________ Date ______________ Class __________

Chapter 10 Knives and Smallwares

PROJECT Culinary Review (continued)
Choose Knives and Smallwares

Step 2 List Preparation Tasks

Directions Examine the recipe you chose. What tasks are involved in preparing the ingredients? List any ingredients that require preparation, as well as the preparation task that must be performed. Use another sheet of paper if you need more room.

Ingredient ______________________________

Preparation ______________________________

____

Ingredient ______________________________

Preparation ______________________________

____

Ingredient ______________________________

Preparation ______________________________

____

Ingredient ______________________________

Preparation ______________________________

____

Ingredient ______________________________

Preparation ______________________________

____

Ingredient ______________________________

Preparation ______________________________

____

Ingredient ______________________________

Preparation ______________________________

____

Name ______________________ Date ______________ Class ____________

Chapter 10 Knives and Smallwares

PROJECT Culinary Review (continued)
Choose Knives and Smallwares

Step 3 Choose the Right Knives and Smallwares

Directions Use the information found in Chapter 10 in your textbook to choose the proper knife or tool to perform the preparation steps you listed in Step 2 of this project. Use another sheet of paper if you need more space.

Ingredient ______________________________

Knife/Smallwares Needed ______________________________

____

Ingredient ______________________________

Knife/Smallwares Needed ______________________________

____

Ingredient ______________________________

Knife/Smallwares Needed ______________________________

____

Ingredient ______________________________

Knife/Smallwares Needed ______________________________

____

Ingredient ______________________________

Knife/Smallwares Needed ______________________________

____

Ingredient ______________________________

Knife/Smallwares Needed ______________________________

____

Ingredient ______________________________

Knife/Smallwares Needed ______________________________

____

For additional culinary projects and study tools, visit this book's Online Learning Center at glencoe.com.

Name ______________________ Date ____________ Class ____________

Chapter 11 Culinary Nutrition

Section 11.1 Nutrition Basics

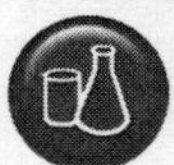

Science Project
Choose Nutritious Menu Options

NCSS C Develop an understanding of matter, energy, and organization in living systems.

Chapter 11

Directions On the line following each of the nutrients, write the effect that nutrient is likely to have on the human body. Then, on the Chef's choice line, list two food sources containing this nutrient that can be a healthful menu option.

1. Proteins ______________________

   Chef's choice for proteins ______________________

2. Carbohydrates ______________________

   Chef's choice for carbohydrates ______________________

3. Fats ______________________

   Chef's choice for monounsaturated fats ______________________

   Chef's choice for polyunsaturated fats ______________________

4. Vitamins A, D, E, and K ______________________

   Chef's choice for Vitamins A, D, E, and K ______________________

5. Vitamins B and C ______________________

   Chef's choice for Vitamins B and C ______________________

Name ____________________ Date __________ Class __________

Chapter 11 Culinary Nutrition

Section 11.2 Meal Planning Guidelines

Culinary Skills Project
Read Food Labels

Directions Review the two product nutrition labels and answer the questions that follow.

REDUCED-FAT MILK

Nutrition Facts
Serving size (245g) 1c
Servings per Container 1

Amount per serving	
Calories 130	Calories from Fat 45
	% Daily Value*
Total Fat 5g	8%
Saturated Fat 3g	15%
Trans Fat 0g	0%
Cholesterol 20mg	8%
Sodium 120mg	5%
Total Carbohydrate 13g	4%
Fiber 0g	0%
Sugars 12g	
Protein 8g	16%
Vitamin A 10% •	Vitamin C 2%
Calcium 50% •	Iron 0%

*Percent Daily Values are based on a 2,000-calorie diet. Your daily values may be higher or lower depending on your calorie needs.

NONFAT MILK

Nutrition Facts
Serving size (249g) 1c
Servings per Container 1

Amount per serving	
Calories 90	Calories from Fat 0
	% Daily Value*
Total Fat 0g	0%
Saturated Fat 0g	0%
Trans Fat 0g	0%
Cholesterol 3mg	0%
Sodium 130mg	5%
Total Carbohydrate 13g	4%
Fiber 0g	0%
Sugars 12g	
Protein 9g	17%
Vitamin A 10% •	Vitamin C 2%
Calcium 25% •	Iron 0%

*Percent Daily Values are based on a 2,000-calorie diet. Your daily values may be higher or lower depending on your calorie needs.

1. What differences do you notice in the nutritional values for these two products?

____

____

2. Why is it important to read and understand food labels in a foodservice operation?

____

____

3. How might the number of servings listed on the label of each product impact the portion size of a menu item?

____

____

Name ______________________ Date ______________ Class ________

Chapter 11 Culinary Nutrition

Section 11.3 Keep Food Nutritious

Culinary Skills Project

Make Nutritious Choices

Chapter 11

Directions Read each example of a common dish. On the lines with each example, explain in a short answer how the dish could be made with less fat, less sodium, and with more nutrients.

1. Fried chicken ______________________

2. Jelly-filled doughnut ______________________

3. Canned chicken stock ______________________

4. Boiled carrots ______________________

5. Ham and cheese sandwich ______________________

Name ______________________ Date ____________ Class ________

Chapter 11 Culinary Nutrition

Study Skills
Staying Healthy

Directions Read the tips for staying healthy. Then, complete the true/false questions below, circling **T** for true or **F** for false.

How to Stay Healthy
Staying healthy will improve your ability to learn. Follow these tips to help maintain your physical, mental, and emotional well-being: • Keep your mind active by reading, solving math problems, working crossword puzzles, or playing games. • Exercise regularly to keep oxygen moving to your brain and throughout your body. • Eat a variety of nutritious foods and avoid junk foods high in sugar, saturated fats, and empty calories. • Keep your stress level low. When you feel stressed, take a few deep breaths, talk to an understanding friend, or go for a walk. • Talk to a parent or other wise adult, a teacher, or a school counselor if you feel depressed. • Stay away from alcohol and drugs of all types, including cigarettes. • Participate in stimulating discussions with friends and family members.

1. A nutrient is a chemical compound that helps the body to carry out its functions. T F
2. Protein is the nutrient that acts as the main source of energy for the body. T F
3. Most plant foods, such as vegetables, grains, nuts, and dried beans, have all of the essential amino acids. T F
4. Too much LDL cholesterol can contribute to heart-related health problems. T F
5. A nutrition label gives information on serving size, calories, and nutrients in food. T F
6. MyPyramid divides food into six food groups. T F
7. Nutritional needs will change throughout a person's life span. T F
8. Overcooking foods will affect their taste and texture, but not their nutritional content. T F
9. Nutrients will no longer be lost from food once it has been cooked. T F
10. Foods can be cooked in less fat when using cast-iron cookware. T F

Name ______________________ Date ____________ Class ________

Chapter 11 Culinary Nutrition

Certification Test Practice

Relieving Test Stress

Directions Read the tips for relieving test stress. Then, complete the multiple-choice test by circling the letter of the question that goes with the correct answer.

Relieve Stress from Test Taking
To relieve test stress, follow these tips: • Practice deep breathing, and visualize yourself succeeding on the test. • Prioritize. Rather than feeling overwhelmed by all the tasks you must complete, decide what you need to deal with at the immediate moment. • Take care of yourself by getting proper rest, eating foods that are healthy for you, and doing things that you enjoy.

1. MyPyramid
- **a.** What is a guide that shows food-related illnesses?
- **b.** What is a chart that shows rates of obesity?
- **c.** What is a guide that shows the recommended food groups?
- **d.** What is an illustration of ancient Egyptian eating habits?

2. Complete protein
- **a.** What is a protein source that contains all essential amino acids?
- **b.** What is a protein source that has been fully digested by the body?
- **c.** What is a nutrient that most people do not need?
- **d.** What is a protein source that does not contain all essential amino acids?

3. Water-soluble vitamins
- **a.** What are vitamins that are stored in the liver?
- **b.** What are vitamins that can build up in the body?
- **c.** What are vitamins that help the body retain water?
- **d.** What are vitamins that must be eaten every day?

4. Direct food additive
- **a.** What is a food additive that has permanent FDA approval?
- **b.** What is a food additive that is purposefully added to enhance or change food?
- **c.** What is a food additive that is added accidentally through a product's packaging method?
- **d.** What is a food additive that is listed on the MyPyramid chart?

5. Dietary Guidelines for Americans
- **a.** What is a source of information on nutritional deficiencies in Americans?
- **b.** What is guide that defines different food groups?
- **c.** What is a source of healthful eating habits for Americans age two and older?
- **d.** What is a guide for healthful cooking methods for Americans?

Name ____________________ Date ____________ Class __________

Chapter 11 Culinary Nutrition

Content and Academic Vocabulary
English Language Arts

NCTE 12 Use language to accomplish individual purposes.

Chapter 11

Directions Unscramble the letters and write the vocabulary term on the lines provided. Then, write the correct terms on the blank lines in the sentences to complete the definitions.

sneesl ____________ **ereaitvnag** ____________

taf ____________ **atirunod** ____________

mleiarn ____________ **utintenr** ____________

raedoyhcrabt ____________ **aldyi eluva** ____________

lero ____________ **ampcti** ____________

1. A ____________ may be either major or trace, but both categories are equally important.
2. The amount of a nutrient that a person needs every day is known as the ____________ of that nutrient.
3. If you ____________ the holding time before serving food, you can minimize the loss of flavor and nutrients.
4. A ____________ is the nutrient that is the body's main source of energy.
5. A person who does not eat meat or other animal-based foods is called a ____________.
6. The ____________ of physical activity is just one of the factors that affect how much energy the body needs.
7. ____________ regulates bodily functions and helps carry some vitamins through the system.
8. Fat and cholesterol play an important ____________ in keeping the body healthy.
9. High blood pressure can ____________ the development of cardiovascular disease.
10. A chemical compound that helps the body carry out its functions is known as a ____________.

Name ______________________ Date __________ Class __________

Chapter 11 Culinary Nutrition

PROJECT

Culinary Review
Evaluate Food Choices

Scenario The U.S. government offers many different ways of evaluating the nutritional value of the food we eat. In this project, you will research information about MyPyramid from the United States Department of Agriculture's (USDA) MyPyramid Web site and use it to analyze the choices on a menu.

Academic Skills You Will Use	Culinary Skills You Will Use
ENGLISH LANGUAGE ARTS **NCTE 3** Apply strategies to interpret texts. **SCIENCE** **NSES C** Develop an understanding of matter, energy, and organization in living systems.	• Nutrition knowledge • Menu determination • Food substitutions

Step 1 Review MyPyramid Food Groups

Directions Follow your teacher's instructions to go online. Visit the MyPyramid Web site at **www.mypyramid.gov**. Review the information on the food groups and how they affect eating habits for most adults. Describe this information in your own words in the space below. Attach another sheet of paper if you need more space.

Name ______________________ Date ____________ Class ____________

Chapter 11 Culinary Nutrition

PROJECT Culinary Review (continued)
Evaluate Food Choices

Step 2 Evaluate the Nutrition of Menu Items

Directions List the ingredients in each menu in their proper food group categories, based on MyPyramid food groups.

Menu A

Appetizer Steamed Vegetable Medley *A cup of gently steamed carrots, broccoli, and squash.*

Entrée Ravioli *A blend of three cheeses—ricotta, mozzarella and Provolone—fried mushrooms, spinach, and tomatoes stuffed in ravioli and covered with tomato and basil sauce.*

Grains ______________________

Vegetables ______________________

Fruits ______________________

Milk ______________________

Meat & Beans ______________________

Oils ______________________

Menu B

Appetizer Steak Noodle Soup *Egg noodles with steak in a cream base.*

Entrée Pork Tenderloin Sandwich *Tender slice of roast pork tenderloin deep fried. Served on whole-wheat bread, with glazed apple dressing.*

Grains ______________________

Vegetables ______________________

Fruits ______________________

Milk ______________________

Meat & Beans ______________________

Oils ______________________

Name ______________ Date ______________ Class ______________

Chapter 11 Culinary Nutrition

PROJECT Culinary Review (continued)
Evaluate Food Choices

Step 3 Suggest Alternatives

Directions Use the MyPyramid and food group information you gathered to answer the questions about Menu A and Menu B.

1. Based on the MyPyramid information you gathered, which menu is more healthful, and why?

____

____

____

____

____

____

2. Using the information on healthful amounts of each food group for most adults, what substitutions might you make for the ingredients in Menu A?

____

____

____

____

____

____

3. Using the information on healthful amounts of each food group for most adults, what substitutions might you make for the ingredients in Menu B?

____

____

____

____

____

____

For additional culinary projects and study tools, visit this book's Online Learning Center at glencoe.com.

Name ____________________ Date ____________ Class ________

Chapter 12 Creating Menus

Section 12.1 The Menu

English Language Arts Project

List Factors that Influence a Menu

> **NCTE 2** Read literature to build an understanding of the human experience.

Directions Read about the seven factors that can influence a menu in Section 12.1 of your textbook. Then, use the lines to help explain in your own words why each factor is important for menu development. The first one is done for you.

1. **Target Customers** Knowing which customers a restaurant wants to target is important because menu dishes, prices, and design style can help attract customers who will want to eat at that restaurant.
2. **Price** ____________________
3. **Type of Food Served** ____________________
4. **Equipment** ____________________
5. **Skill of Workers** ____________________
6. **Geography and Culture** ____________________
7. **Eating Trends** ____________________

Name ______________________ Date ______________ Class ________

Chapter 12 Creating Menus

Section 12.2 Menu Planning and Design

NCTE 5 Use different writing process elements to communicate effectively.

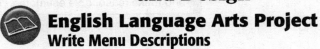

English Language Arts Project

Write Menu Descriptions

Directions In the chart, write a menu description for each food item listed. Use the truth-in-menu guidelines in Chapter 12 of your textbook for guidance.

Menu Item	Description
Potato Skins	
Steakhouse Noodle Soup	
Grilled Chicken Salad	
Turkey and Dressing	
Cheddar Cheese Mashed Potatoes	
Apple Pie	
Raspberry Lemonade	

Chapter 12

Name ____________________ Date ____________ Class ____________

Chapter 12 Creating Menus

Section 12.3 Pricing Menu Items

Mathematics Project
Compare Pricing Methods

NCTM Number and Operations Compute fluently and make reasonable estimates.

Directions Michelle would like to add a combo meal with a grilled chicken sandwich, small green salad, and a beverage to her lunch menu. The total food cost of the combo meal is $3.29. Answer the following questions, and remember to show your work.

1. If Michelle's restaurant had sales of $240,000 and total food costs of $90,000 last year, calculate the price of the combo meal using the factor method.

2. If Michelle wants her food cost percentage to be 30%, calculate the price of the combo meal using the markup-on-cost method.

3. If Michelle expects to serve 2,500 customers a month, and her monthly overhead costs (including an allowance for profit) are $9,500, calculate the price of the combo meal using the contribution margin method.

4. Michelle's local competitors charge the following amounts for a similar combo meal:

Al's	Bubba's	Carl's	Debbie's	Emma's	Frankie's	Gina's
$9.95	$7.50	$12.85	$13.75	$8.95	$10.00	$11.50

a) If Michelle wants her combo meal to be priced at the average of her competitors' prices, what should the price be?

b) If Michelle wants her combo meal to be 10% more expensive than the average of her competitors, what should the price be?

c) If Michelle wants to be 5% cheaper than her cheapest competitor, what should the price be?

Name ______________________ Date __________ Class __________

Chapter 12 Creating Menus

Study Skills
Balancing School and Social Life

Directions Read the tips for balancing school and a social life. Then, use the prompt to write two paragraphs about how you might fit in working at a foodservice establishment with your other responsibilities.

How to Balance School and Social Life
• Schedule time with friends. Socializing and having fun are important parts of life. • Identify your priorities, and create a schedule that reflects them. • Look for activities, such as school clubs, that allow you to combine academic enrichment with socializing. • Get involved in activities only because you want to, not because you think you should or because someone else wants you to. • Do not overdo it. Make sure your activities will fit into your schedule. • Ideally, you should participate in a few long-term activities. These will demonstrate to colleges and prospective employers that you are able to commit, and that you are interested in the world around you. • Some activities cost money, so make sure the ones you choose will fit into your budget or your family's budget.

Write two paragraphs explaining how you might fit in working at a foodservice establishment with your other responsibilities.

____

____

____

____

____

____

____

____

____

____

____

____

Name ______________________ Date ______________ Class ____________

Chapter 12 Creating Menus

Certification Test Practice

Practicing Time Management

Directions Read these tips about time management during written tests. Then, answer the questions.

Tips for Test Time Management
• Before you begin the test, read the test directions carefully to make sure you understand exactly what you are being asked to do. • Take note of the actual number of questions and the type of questions. This can help you budget the time you will need to answer each question. For example, a short-answer question may take more time for you to answer than a multiple-choice question. • If you do not know the answer to a particular question, skip that question and move on to the next question. • If you are unable to think of the correct answer to a question, brainstorm words and phrases that are related to that question and write them down. Brainstorming can prompt you to remember information. • After you have reached the end of the test, go back to the questions you have skipped and mark an answer. Even if your answer is a guess, you may have a chance of getting the question right.

Chapter 12

Reading Check

1. What are some strategies you can use to budget your time during a test?

____

____

2. What should you do if you are unable to think of the correct answer to a question?

____

____

Practice

3. Using a clock, allow yourself a maximum of 10 minutes to write at least 200 words explaining how a creative menu can help a business be more profitable. Use complete sentences, and use another sheet of paper if you need more room.

____

____

____

____

Name ______________________ Date ____________ Class ________

Chapter 12 Creating Menus

Content and Academic Vocabulary

English Language Arts

NCTE 12 Use language to accomplish individual purposes.

Directions Use the right column of the chart to list the best vocabulary term from the list. Then, write a sentence in the left column using the word. The first one is done for you. You will not use all the terms.

Content Vocabulary		Academic Vocabulary	
garnish entrée fixed menu accompaniment extender	operating cost factor method cycle menu	entice upscale	guide dictate

To attract **1.** The new menu was designed to **entice** diners with its colorful descriptions.	entice
Anything that is a cost of doing business **2.**	
A system that uses a pricing scale based on a percentage of the food and nonfood costs needed to operate a restaurant successfully **3.**	
For more affluent customers; fashionable **4.**	
An edible food that is placed on or around food to add color or flavor **5.**	
A menu that offers the same dishes every day for a long period of time **6.**	
Any type of main dish **7.**	

Chapter 12

Name ______________________ Date ____________ Class ____________

Chapter 12 Creating Menus

PROJECT Culinary Review
Research Menu Types

Scenario The type of menu that a restaurant chooses can affect how customers will react to the business. In this project, you will define menu types, find examples of those menu types, and answer questions about them. You will also be asked to make changes to one of the menus.

Academic Skills You Will Use	Culinary Skills You Will Use
ENGLISH LANGUAGE ARTS **NCTE 3** Apply strategies to interpret texts. **SOCIAL STUDIES** **NCSS V C Individuals, Groups, and Institutions** Describe the various forms institutions take, and explain how they develop and change over time.	• Menu knowledge • Food trends • Customer service

Chapter 12

Step 1 Define Menu Types

Directions Follow the directions given. Follow your teacher's instructions to use the Internet.

Define the following menu types, in your own words:

Fixed menu ____

____

____

Cycle menu ____

____

____

Á la carte menu ____

____

____

Table d'hôte menu ____

____

____

Use the Internet to locate and print a sample of one of each type of menu listed above. Attach the samples to this sheet.

Name ____________________ Date ______________ Class ____________

Chapter 12 Creating Menus

PROJECT Culinary Review (continued)
Research Menu Types

Step 2 Evaluate Each Menu

Directions Evaluate each of the menus you printed by answering the following questions for each.

1. Who are the target customers for each menu?

A. ______________________________

B. ______________________________

C. ______________________________

D. ______________________________

2. What is the price range of each menu?

A. ______________________________

B. ______________________________

C. ______________________________

D. ______________________________

3. How does each menu's design reflect its target customers?

A. ______________________________

B. ______________________________

C. ______________________________

D. ______________________________

4. What eating trends are reflected in each menu?

A. ______________________________

B. ______________________________

C. ______________________________

D. ______________________________

Chapter 12

Name ______________________ Date ____________ Class ________

Chapter 12 Creating Menus

PROJECT Culinary Review (continued)
Research Menu Types

Step 3 Change a Menu

Directions Choose one of the menus you have evaluated. Imagine that you are the owner of that restaurant. You want to target a different market, and so you must change some elements of your menu. Write a short essay to discuss who the new target customers are, and what specific things you would do to change the menu to attract them.

Chapter 12

For additional culinary projects and study tools, visit this book's Online Learning Center at **glencoe.com**.

Name ______________________ Date ______________ Class ____________

Chapter 13 Using Standardized Recipes

Section 13.1 Standardized Recipe Basics

Culinary Skills Project
Identify Parts of a Recipe

Directions Identify the parts of the recipe. Write your answers in the space provided.

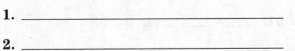

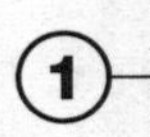

Southern Vegetable Soup

YIELD: 10 SERVINGS
SERVING SIZE: 8 OZ.

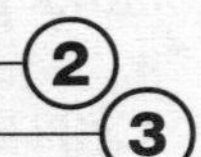

Ingredients

2 oz.	Salt pork, cut into a small dice
10 oz.	Beef, bottom round, cut into small cubes
8 oz.	Canned peeled tomatoes, drained, seeded, and chopped
3½ qts.	Beef stock, heated to a boil
2 oz.	Frozen green beans
2 oz.	Red beans, cooked
4 oz.	Onions, peeled and diced brunoise
3 oz.	Celery stalks, washed, trimmed, and diced brunoise
6 oz.	Green cabbage, washed, cored, and chiffonade
3 oz.	Carrots, washed, peeled, and diced brunoise
2 oz.	Frozen corn kernels
2 oz.	Frozen okra, sliced
2 oz.	Zucchini, washed, trimmed, and cut in ½-in. dice
to taste	Salt and black pepper

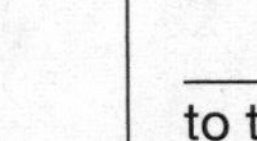

Method of Preparation

1. In a large marmite, place the salt pork, and render the fat, stirring frequently until browned. Add the beef, reduce the heat, and sauté until browned.
2. Add the tomatoes, and sauté for another 2 minutes.
3. Add the boiling stock, and simmer until the meat is slightly firm in texture.
4. Add all other ingredients, and continue to simmer until vegetables are tender.
5. Season to taste and serve immediately in preheated cups, or hold at 135°F (57°C) or above. Reheat to 165°F (74°C) for 15 seconds.

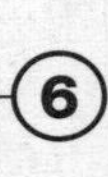

1. ______________________

2. ______________________

3. ______________________

4. ______________________

5. ______________________

6. ______________________

Name ______________ Date ______________ Class ______________

Chapter 13 Using Standardized Recipes

Section 13.2 Recipe Measurement and Conversion

NCTM Measurement Apply appropriate techniques, tools, and formulas to determine measurements.

Mathematics Project
Convert Equivalents

Directions Convert the following equivalents. Write your answers on the blanks provided.

1. 32 T. = ______ c.
2. 12 pts. = ______ gal.
3. 4 pts. = ______ qts.
4. 6 tsp. = ______ Tbsp.
5. 24 oz. = ______ lbs.
6. ½ c. = ______ oz.
7. ¼ c. = ______ oz.
8. 4 c. = ______ gal.
9. 4 qts. = ______ gal.
10. 8 c. = ______ gal.
11. 4 oz. = ______ tsp.
12. 24 tsp. = ______ Tbsp.
13. 1 pt. = ______ qt.
14. 1¾ qts. = ______ c.
15. 1 c. = ______ Tbsp.
16. 1 c. = ______ oz.
17. 6 lbs. = ______ c.
18. ¼ c. = ______ Tbsp.
19. 1 qt. = ______ oz.
20. 6 c. = ______ oz.
21. 1 lb. = ______ oz.
22. 1 Tbsp. = ______ tsp.
23. 9 Tbsp. = ______ tsp.
24. 3 qts. = ______ pts.
25. ⅛ c. = ______ oz.
26. ⅛ c. = ______ Tbsp.
27. 4 qts. = ______ gal.
28. ⅞ c. = ______ oz.
29. ¾ c. = ______ Tbsp.
30. 1 c. = ______ pt.
31. ½ c. = ______ oz.
32. 22 c. = ______ qts.

Chapter 13

Name ____________________ Date ____________ Class ________

Chapter 13 Using Standardized Recipes

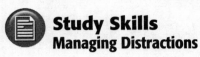

Study Skills
Managing Distractions

Directions Read the tips on managing distractions. Then, apply the tips as you read Chapter 13. Answer the questions.

Tips to Manage Distractions
• Find a quiet place to study. Reading comprehension usually decreases in relation to the amount of sound in the room. • If you cannot eliminate noise from the room, try blocking it out with white noise. White noise is dull background noise; for example, try turning on a fan. Your mind will get used to the white noise and tune it out. • Certain kinds of music have the same effect as white noise. Easy listening or classical music can sometimes keep you from getting distracted. • Eliminate worries, thoughts, and daydreams that keep you from concentrating.

1. Did your reading comprehension improve by finding a quieter place to read? Why, or why not?

____

____

2. Did your comprehension improve by creating white noise while you read? Why, or why not?

____

____

3. Did your comprehension improve by listening to music? Why, or why not?

____

____

4. Did your comprehension improve by eliminating worries and daydreams? Why, or why not?

____

____

5. What strategies worked best for you? Explain.

____

____

Chapter 13

Name ______________________ Date ____________ Class __________

Chapter 13 Using Standardized Recipes

Certification Test Practice
Eliminating Test Jitters

Directions Read the tips. Then, answer the questions about Chapter 13.

Tips to Eliminate Test Jitters
• Having jitters, or being nervous, before and during a test is normal. • Remember that this is only a test. Each test is important, but it is not the only test on which your grade depends. • When you feel nervous, take a deep breath. Clear your mind as you hold your breath. Exhale gently. • Rest is important. Get plenty of sleep the night before a test. • Dress in layers. If you get hot, you can remove a layer, or you can put one on if you get cold. Being comfortable during a test is important.

Chapter 13

1. What benefits will you get from carefully following a recipe?

____

____

2. What is an ingredient list?

____

____

3. Common examples of weight measurements are:

- ○ Celsius and Fahrenheit
- ○ gallons and quarts
- ○ ounces and pounds
- ○ inches and feet

4. How do you find the conversion factor for a recipe?

____

____

5. How would you deal with problems that arise when testing a converted recipe?

____

____

Name ______________________ Date ______________ Class ____________

Chapter 13 Using Standardized Recipes

Content and Academic Vocabulary
English Language Arts

NCTE 12 Use language to accomplish individual purposes.

Directions Find and circle 10 vocabulary and academic terms in the word-search puzzle. Terms appear vertically, diagonally, and horizontally.

Content Vocabulary		Academic Vocabulary
recipe	electronic scale	hallmark
quality control	count	precise
yield	shrinkage	alter
formula		

w	o	c	z	b	n	v	p	u	y	c	l	s	a	t
c	w	o	m	e	e	f	o	r	m	u	l	a	m	x
k	o	u	u	n	c	p	e	i	q	g	s	a	p	n
l	z	u	w	p	r	e	c	i	s	e	l	e	y	c
m	r	t	n	j	e	m	o	d	e	l	y	v	u	o
a	d	r	c	t	c	n	a	t	l	c	e	h	a	d
s	l	i	b	d	i	l	i	b	e	r	a	t	s	r
v	t	t	s	o	p	s	r	e	g	a	m	e	l	e
b	f	g	e	c	e	e	i	r	r	y	s	o	m	h
e	l	r	m	r	i	n	g	o	o	v	r	e	a	p
q	u	a	l	i	t	y	c	o	n	t	r	o	l	a
u	u	m	e	l	e	v	l	w	a	f	q	p	k	r
l	p	y	o	a	m	q	e	i	g	e	a	r	k	e
e	l	e	c	t	r	o	n	i	c	s	c	a	l	e
y	e	o	p	b	c	o	p	v	e	e	b	c	w	t
i	i	n	q	o	o	d	h	a	n	y	w	e	e	i
p	l	e	e	s	h	r	i	n	k	a	g	e	e	n
e	e	d	l	t	o	p	r	a	p	p	t	o	r	g
n	c	l	v	d	q	k	a	k	w	l	d	c	e	e
e	t	e	k	s	h	a	l	l	m	a	r	k	p	t

Chapter 13

Name ______________________ Date ______________ Class __________

Chapter 13 Using Standardized Recipes

PROJECT Culinary Review
Use Commercial Scales

Scenario Using a commercial scale properly is vital to making recipes and formulas come out correctly. A foodservice worker must know how to use all types of scales. In this project, you will describe the different types of scales, explain how they are used, and use them to weigh different food items.

Academic Skills You Will Use	Culinary Skills You Will Use
ENGLISH LANGUAGE ARTS **NCTE 4** Use written language to communicate effectively. **MATHEMATICS** **NCTM Measurement** Apply appropriate techniques, tools, and formulas to determine measurements.	• Weighing and measuring • Measuring tool use

Step 1 Identify Professional Scales

Directions Identify the following scales, and describe them in the space given below.

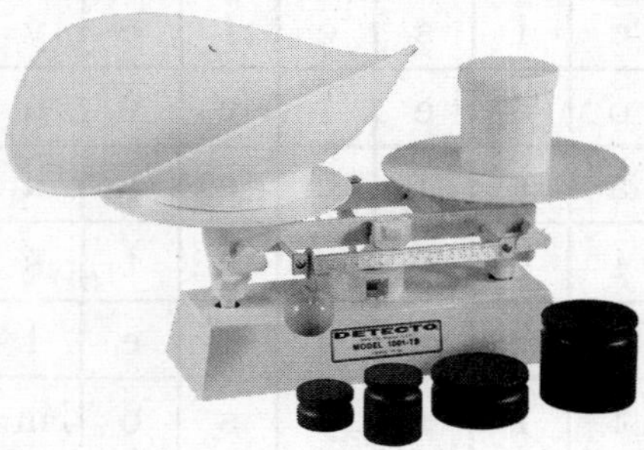

A. Type of Scale: ______________________

Purpose: ______________________

____

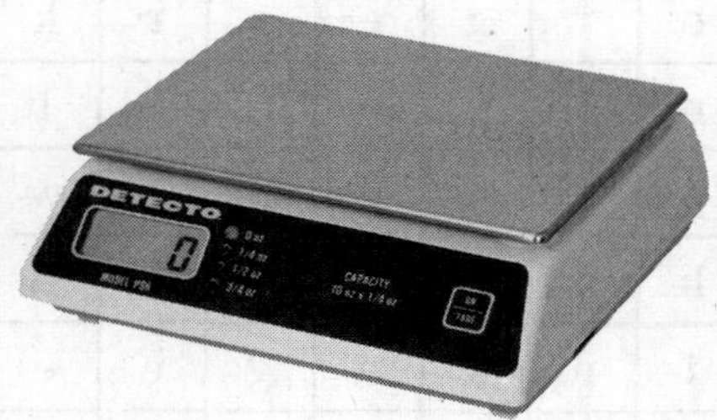

B. Type of Scale: ______________________

Purpose: ______________________

____

Chapter 13

Name ____________ Date ____________ Class ____________

Chapter 13 Using Standardized Recipes

PROJECT Culinary Review (continued)
Use Commercial Scales

Step 2 Describe Weighing Methods

Directions Use your textbook and other resources to find methods of using both types of scales. Write out the methods you find on the lines provided.

Scale A: ____________

Scale B: ____________

Chapter 13

Name ____________________ Date __________ Class __________

Chapter 13 Using Standardized Recipes

PROJECT Culinary Review (continued)
Use Commercial Scales

Step 3 Weigh Ingredients

Directions Follow your teacher's instructions to form groups. Use the two different types of scales to weigh the following ingredients, and answer the questions.

1. Weigh 1 pound of potatoes. How many potatoes do you have? __________
2. Measure 2 tablespoons of salt. How much does the salt weigh? __________
3. Measure 2 tablespoons of garlic powder. How much does the garlic powder weigh? __________
4. Measure 2 tablespoons of dried basil. How much does the dried basil weigh? __________
5. Weigh one bunch of celery. How much does the celery weigh? __________
6. Measure 1 cup of packed brown sugar. How much does the sugar weigh? __________
7. Measure 1 cup of flour. How much does the flour weigh? __________
8. Measure 1 cup of granulated sugar. How much does it weigh? __________

What can you determine about weight and measurement from this experiment? Explain your answer.

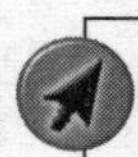

For additional culinary projects and study tools, visit this book's Online Learning Center at glencoe.com.

Name ______________________ Date ______________ Class ______________

Chapter 14 Cost Control Techniques

Section 14.1 Calculating Food Costs

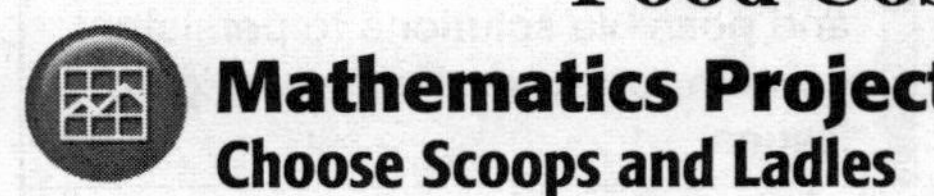

NCTM Measurement Understand measureable attributes of objects and the units, systems, and processes of measurement.

Directions Read each of the word problems. Write your answers to the questions on the blanks provided. Use the chart of scoops and ladles to help you find the answers.

Scoops	Ladles
#8 scoop = 8 Tbsp. (½ c.)	#1 ladle = 1 oz.
#12 scoop = 5 ⅓ Tbsp. (⅓ c.)	#2 ladle = 2 oz.
#16 scoop = 4 Tbsp. (¼ c.)	#3 ladle = 3 oz.
#20 scoop = 3 Tbsp.	#4 ladle = 4 oz.
#24 scoop = 2 ⅔ Tbsp.	#6 ladle = 6 oz.
#30 scoop = 2 Tbsp.	#8 ladle = 8 oz.
#40 scoop = 1 ⅔ Tbsp.	
#60 scoop = 1 Tbsp.	
#70 scoop = 1 ½ – 2 tsp.	

_____ **1.** A baker made 2 quarts of chocolate pudding. A serving is ½ cup. What scoop should you use, and how many servings will it yield?

_____ **2.** A cook has made 1½ gallons of sauce. How many servings will the sauce yield if a #6 ladle is used?

_____ **3.** A caterer prepared 2 quarts of a sauerkraut ball mixture. A sauerkraut ball equals ½ tablespoon. What scoop should you use, and how many sauerkraut balls will it yield?

_____ **4.** How many servings are there in 3 quarts of garlic mashed potatoes if each customer is given two #12 scoops?

_____ **5.** A cook prepared 4½ quarts of chicken casserole. A serving is ⅔ cup. What scoop should you use, and how many servings will it yield?

_____ **6.** A banquet is to be served to 120 people. If a #2 ladle is used for the gravy, how much gravy should be prepared?

Name _______________ Date _______ Class _______

Chapter 14 Cost Control Techniques

Section 14.2 Managing Food Cost Factors

NCSS IX D Global Connections
Analyze the causes, consequences, and possible solutions to persistent, contemporary, and emerging global issues.

Social Studies Project

Assess Regional, National, and Global Factors

Directions Research the effects of supply and demand on food supplies. What regional, national, and global factors might affect the price and availability of different foods? Use the space provided to write a short essay on your findings.

Chapter 14

Name ______________________ Date ____________ Class __________

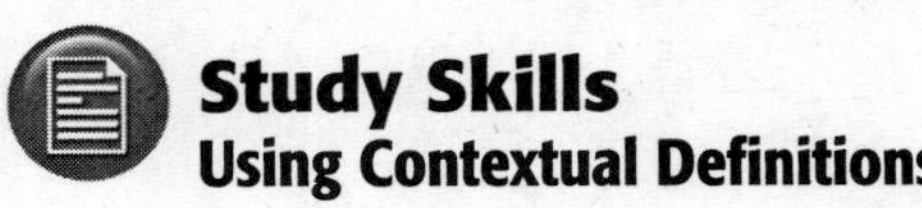

Chapter 14 Cost Control Techniques

Study Skills
Using Contextual Definitions

Directions Read the following tips and the passage about food costs. Then, write your own definitions for the numbered terms based on contextual clues in the passage.

Tips for Using Contextual Definitions
Contextual definitions will help you understand the meaning of words you do not know as well as ideas that are hard to comprehend. Look for clues from the larger content of the text to help you figure out the meaning of unknown words or ideas. To read using contextual definitions, follow these steps: • As you read a passage, circle unfamiliar words. • Reread the sentence in which the unfamiliar word appears. • Focus on what you do understand in the sentence. It may help to reread the sentences before and after the one in which the unfamiliar word appears. • In your own words, state the meaning of the sentence. You may know only part of the meaning. State as much as you can. • Based on the meaning of the sentence, guess what the unfamiliar word means.

Types of Food Costs
Food cost is the total dollar amount spent by a foodservice operation to purchase food and beverages needed to prepare menu items intended for sale. Food costs include produce, meats, poultry, seafood, baking goods, and other food items that are needed to prepare a recipe. Beverage cost is the total dollar amount spent by the foodservice operation to acquire all the ingredients needed to make different beverages. Beverage costs usually represent 15 to 20 percent of money earned through beverage sales. Labor cost is the cost of paying employees wages, salaries, and benefits. Overhead costs include all other expenses for operating the business. The combination of labor costs and overhead costs are termed operating expenses.

1. intended ______________________________

2. acquire ______________________________

3. represent ______________________________

4. termed ______________________________

Chapter 14

Name ______________________ Date ______________ Class __________

Chapter 14 Cost Control Techniques

Certification Test Practice
Organizing Study Groups

Directions Read the tips for organizing study groups. Then, take the sentence completion test. Write in short answers to complete the sentences relating to Chapter 14.

Tips to Organize a Study Group
Studying in a group can be an effective way to prepare for tests. To organize a study group: • Invite three to five students to form a study group. • Invite students who share a desire to practice good study habits, learn material well, and succeed on tests. • Meet in a place and at a time that is convenient for everyone in the study group, such as in the school library at the end of the school day. • Plan on a meeting regularly for at least an hour each time. • During meetings, take short breaks to recharge your minds and help the group to stay focused.

1. The three guidelines that can help you control portions are ______________________
____

2. Buying food in bulk is effective so long as ______________________
____

3. Raw yield tests are used on ______________________
____

4. The four types of products a foodservice business can purchase are ______________________
____
____

5. The relationship between a vendor and a foodservice business must be based on ______
____

6. Inventory should include ______________________
____
____

Chapter 14

Name ______________________ Date ____________ Class ________

Chapter 14 Cost Control Techniques

Content and Academic Vocabulary
English Language Arts

NCTE 12 Use language to accomplish individual purposes.

Directions Write the vocabulary term or terms that best completes each sentence. The first one is done for you. You will not use all the terms.

Content Vocabulary		Academic Vocabulary
specification	as-purchased (AP) price	confirm
unit cost	sales cycle	deteriorate
product yield	parstock	implement
requisition	cost per portion	aspect
Q factor	trim loss	

1. Marybelle had to ___confirm___ delivery of the fresh produce each day.

2. The restaurant's manager determined the ____________ by dividing the recipe cost by the number of portions he planned for the day.

3. Filippi filled out a(n) ____________ each time he had to take supplies out of storage.

4. The longer a food product is stored, the more its quality may ____________.

5. To find out how much it costs to make one recipe, your must convert the bulk price, called the ____________, to the ____________, the cost of each item.

6. After chef Romero finished preparing his entrees, he calculated the ____________, the amount of food product left.

7. A foodservice manager must know how much of each product the chef expects to use to prepare menu items for a given ____________, the period of time between supply deliveries.

8. It is important to know how much ____________ a restaurant will need from one supply delivery to another.

9. Each food product needs to be purchased according to a(n) ____________ that describes the product.

10. The ____________ is the questionable ingredient factor that is difficult to measure.

Chapter 14

Name ________________________ Date ____________ Class __________

Chapter 14 Cost Control Techniques

PROJECT Culinary Review
Calculate Food Costs

Scenario A foodservice business must keep food costs in mind as it plans menus. If food costs get out of control, a business will lose money. In this project, you will calculate the unit price, perform a raw yield test, and find a yield percentage for several ingredients.

Academic Skills You Will Use	Culinary Skills You Will Use
MATHEMATICS **NCTM Measurement** Apply appropriate techniques, tools, and formulas to determine measurements. **NCTM Number and Operations** Compute fluently and make reasonable estimates.	• Food preparation skills • Weighing and measuring • Cost control techniques

Step 1 Calculate Unit Price

Directions Complete the Unit Cost chart by calculating the unit price for each ingredient and recording the results in the far-right column.

Unit Cost		
Food Product	**As-Purchased Price**	**Unit Price**
Carrots	1 pound/$0.95	/ounce
Apples	6 pounds/$7.85	/ounce
Celery	1 pound/$1.25	/ounce
Oranges	1 pound/$0.89	/ounce
Shredded cheese	5 pounds/$10.25	/ounce
Milk	1 gallon/$2.29	/fluid ounce
Onions, whole fresh	12 pounds/$10.98	/ounce
Stew meat, 2-inch cubed	10 pounds/$28.90	/ounce
Cabbage	50 pounds/$34.95	/ounce
Bananas	4 pounds/$0.79	/ounce

Chapter 14

Name ______________________ Date ____________ Class ____________

Chapter 14 Cost Control Techniques

PROJECT Culinary Review (continued)
Calculate Food Costs

Step 2 Perform a Raw Yield Test

Directions Follow your teacher's direction to choose one or more of the following foods from your chart: carrots (10), apples (4), celery (1 bunch), oranges (4), cabbage (1 head), onions (4 medium), bananas (4). Complete the steps to perform the raw yield test.

A. Weigh the food on a food scale to get the AP (as-purchased) weight. Record this figure in the third column of the chart for Step 3.

B. Clean the food and trim off any unusable parts.

C. Weigh the unusable parts (trim loss). Record this figure in the fourth column of the chart for Step 3.

D. Subtract the trim loss weight from the AP weight to find the yield weight. Use this formula: **AP weight − trim loss weight = yield weight**. Record this figure in the fifth column of the chart for Step 3. Show your work in the space provided.

AP weight − trim loss weight = yield weight

Chapter 14

Name ______________________ Date ______________ Class ______________

Chapter 14 Cost Control Techniques

PROJECT Culinary Review (continued)
Calculate Food Costs

Step 3 Calculate Yield Percentage

Directions Follow the direction to calculate yield percentage using the figures you recorded from Step 2. Then, record your results in the sixth column in the chart.

A. Divide the yield weight for each food by the AP weight to find the yield percentage for each food. Use this formula: **yield weight ÷ AP weight = yield percentage**. Show your work in the space provided.

yield weight ÷ AP weight = yield percentage

Raw Yield Percentage					
Item	**Amount**	**AP Weight**	**Trim Loss Weight**	**Yield Weight**	**Yield Percentage**
Carrots	10				
Apples	4				
Celery	1 bunch				
Oranges	4				
Cabbage	1 head				
Onions	4 medium				
Bananas	4				

For additional culinary projects and study tools, visit this book's Online Learning Center at glencoe.com.

Chapter 14

Name ______________________ Date ______________ Class ___________

COMPETITIVE EVENTS PRACTICE

Make a Nutritious Dip

Directions Follow your teacher's instructions to form competition teams of two to four people. Each team will research a nutritious alternative to fatty dips, and will make a dip based on their research. Special attention should be paid to fat content and flavor.

Judging
In this competition, you will be judged on:
• The fat content in your dip • The appearance and flavor of your dip • The sanitation procedures you follow • The cleanliness of your workspace

Preparation Phase

1. Write a description of the dip your team chooses to make. Turn in a copy of your description to your teacher.

   ____

   ____

   ____

2. Prepare your workspace for competition. During preparation:
   - Retrieve all necessary equipment and tools
   - Observe all safety and sanitation procedures
   - Keep foods at the proper temperature
   - Use a sanitizing solution to clean your workspace before beginning

   Do not prepare any part of the dip at this time.

Cooking Phase

1. Make your dip, following the description you created. You must make two portions of your dip—one to be tasted, and one for presentation. There should not be a visible difference between the two dips. You will have 30 minutes to make your dips.

2. Bring both dips to the tasting area designated by your teacher when they are completed and ready for judging, or at the end of the time period. Display your dips with the dip description you wrote earlier.

COMPETITIVE EVENTS PRACTICE (continued)

Competitive Events Review

Once the competition has been completed, write a short essay on the experience of creating a nutritious, low-fat dip. Which ingredients did you choose as a base for your dip, and why? How did you add flavor to your dip? What would you have done differently the next time?

Chapter 15 Cooking Techniques

Section 15.1 How Cooking Alters Food

NSES B Develop an understanding of the interactions of energy and matter.

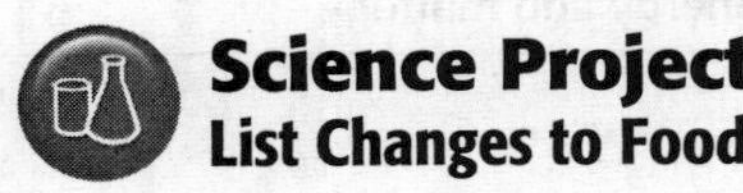

Science Project
List Changes to Food

Directions Use Chapter 15 in your textbook as reference to describe five types of changes that you could expect to take place in chicken that is baked from its raw form to its finished state. Explain how the cooking process makes these changes occur.

1. Nutritive value

____

____

____

2. Texture

____

____

____

3. Color

____

____

____

4. Aroma

____

____

____

5. Flavor

____

____

____

Name ______________________ Date ____________ Class ________

Chapter 15 Cooking Techniques

Section 15.2 Dry Cooking Techniques

NSES B Develop an understanding of the interactions of energy and matter.

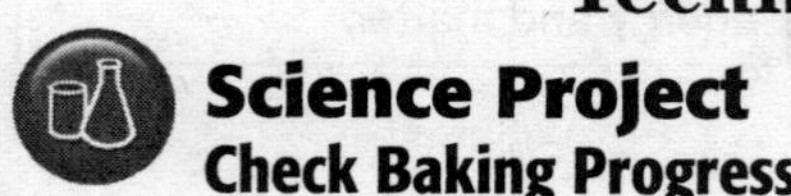

Science Project
Check Baking Progress

Directions Follow your teacher's instructions to form groups. As a group, bake a medium-size potato. Record your observations of the potato's progress every 8 to 10 minutes. Write the exact time of each report. Remove the potato from the oven when you think it is done and record the time. Cut open the potato. Did you undercook or overcook it? Compare your results with those of your classmates and summarize. Use another sheet of paper for your summary if you need more space.

Potato Baking Progress		
Stage	**Starting Time of Stage**	**Observations**
Place in oven		
First check		
Second check		
Third check		
Remove from oven		

Summary of Class Results

____

____

____

____

____

Chapter 15

Name ________________________ Date ______________ Class ________

Chapter 15 Cooking Techniques

Section 15.3 Moist Cooking Techniques

Culinary Skills Project
Make Tomato Concassé

Directions Follow your teacher's directions to form teams. Working in teams, practice using the moist cooking techniques needed to prepare tomato concassé. Once you have finished, answer the questions.

Make Tomato Concassé
1. Gather a 1-quart saucepan, a 1-quart bowl of ice water, a tomato, a slotted spoon, a paring knife, a chef's knife, and a cutting board. 2. Set the saucepan on the burner. Rinse the tomato. Place the tomato in the saucepan. Fill the saucepan with enough water to cover the tomato. 3. Remove the tomato. Let the water begin to heat until it comes to a simmer. 4. Remove the stem and cut an "X" in the bottom of the tomato. 5. Put the tomato in the saucepan. Blanch the tomato for 15 to 30 seconds. 6. Remove the tomato from the simmering water. 7. Plunge the tomato into the ice water. This is called the shocking process. 8. Remove the skin from the tomato. 9. Cut the tomato in half crosswise. 10. Gently squeeze out the seeds, and dice the tomato. This is the final product.

1. How do you think blanching and shocking affected the process?

____

____

____

2. Why would a chef want to prepare tomatoes in this way?

____

____

____

3. In what dishes might a chef want to use tomato concassé?

____

____

____

Chapter 15

Name ____________________ Date ____________ Class ____________

Chapter 15 Cooking Techniques

Study Skills
Determining Your Learning Style

Directions Read about the different learning styles. Then, answer the questions.

Types of Learning Styles
People learn in different ways. For example: • Auditory learners learn best by listening, such as to a teacher's lecture. • Visual learners learn best by seeing, such as reading or viewing a demonstration. • Tactile learners learn best by touching or doing, such as writing or performing an action. • Interpersonal learners learn best by sharing, comparing, and cooperating. Experiment with different styles. After determining your learning style, you can study more effectively in less time.

1. If you are a tactile learner, how could you become better organized?

____

____

2. If you are an auditory learner, how could you better prepare for a test?

____

____

3. If you are a visual learner, how could you remember what you hear while listening to a class discussion?

____

____

4. If you are a tactile learner, how could you remember what you hear while listening to a class discussion?

____

____

5. If you are an interpersonal learner, how could you best prepare for a test?

____

____

Name ________________ Date ____________ Class ________

Chapter 15 Cooking Techniques

Certification Test Practice
Reviewing After a Test

Directions Read the tips for what to do after a test. Then, complete the test, which combines multiple-choice, true/false, fill-in-the-blank, and short-answer questions.

What to Do After a Test

- Fight the urge to turn in your test as soon as you have finished. Use any extra time to check your work.
- Make any changes you think are important.
- Consider whether any questions you answered later in the test provide information that might help you answer questions you were not sure of earlier.
- Evaluate your performance on the test. Think about what you can do to perform better on future tests.
- When you get your corrected test back, look it over to make sure there are no grading mistakes.
- Look over the answers you got wrong. Make sure you understand why they were wrong. Ask your teacher for clarification if you are unsure.
- Save the test for future study. Cumulative final exams often contain questions from previous tests.

Fill in the bubble next to the answer that best completes the statement.

1. Some people might choose to steam vegetables because

○ it is a gentle dry cooking method.
○ minimal nutrients will be lost in cooking.
○ no nutrients will be lost in cooking.
○ water is an inexpensive cooking medium.

Use a content vocabulary term from Chapter 15 to fill in the blank.

2. When you force foods to stand up to heat, you ____________ them to chemical changes.

Circle the appropriate answer.

3. Placing meat on a metal rod and slowly rotating it over a heat source is called searing. T F

Write a short answer for the question.

4. What is the difference between blanching and parboiling?

____

____

Chapter 15

Name ______________________ Date ______________ Class ______________

Chapter 15 Cooking Techniques

Content and Academic Vocabulary
English Language Arts

NCTE 12 Use language to accomplish individual purposes.

Directions Match the vocabulary terms to their definitions. Write in the letter corresponding to each term next to the definition that matches it.

a. dry cooking technique	_____	the process that occurs when liquids boil
b. moist cooking technique	_____	to expose
c. coagulate	_____	to change from a liquid or semiliquid state to a drier, solid state
d. caramelization	_____	the time it takes for the fat or oil to return to temperature after the food has been submerged
e. carryover cooking	_____	fragile
f. recovery time	_____	to decrease the volume of
g. convection	_____	the process of cooking sugar to a high temperatures
h. blanching	_____	uses oil, fat, hot air radiation, or metal to transfer heat
i. reduce	_____	uses liquid instead of oil to create the heat energy needed to cook food
j. braising	_____	cooking that takes place after you remove something from its heat source
k. deglaze	_____	using the boiling method to partially cook food
l. subject	_____	to add a small amount of liquid to a pan to loosen bits of food after searing or sautéing
m. delicate	_____	a long, slow cooking process
n. extracted	_____	drawn out

Chapter 15

Chapter 15 Cooking Techniques

PROJECT Culinary Review
Evaluate Food Browning

Scenario How important is browning to the flavor and texture of foods? In this project, you will cook three different foods, evaluate their flavor and texture, and describe the importance of the results for a foodservice business.

Academic Skills You Will Use	Culinary Skills You Will Use
ENGLISH LANGUAGE ARTS **NCTE 5** Use different writing process elements to communicate effectively. **SCIENCE** **NSES B** Develop an understanding of chemical reactions.	• Dry cooking skills • Food safety and sanitation • Sensory evaluation

Step 1 Cook Three Foods

Directions Follow your teacher's instructions to form teams. As a team, choose three food items from the list. Then, complete the cooking steps for each food.

- Mushrooms
- Broccoli
- Carrots
- Pears
- Pork chops
- Fish
- Chicken
- Onions
- Bell peppers
- Apples
- Ham
- Sirloin tips

Cooking Steps:

1. Place a small amount of oil in a shallow pan or wok.
2. Heat the pan until you see ripples in the oil.
3. Add one food item to the pan. Note your start time, and mark it on the chart for Step 2.
4. Cook the food item until it browns, observing the browning process. Note your stop time, and mark it on the chart for Step 2.
5. Repeat Cooking Step 3 and Cooking Step 4 for each food item, recording your start and stop times on the chart on the next page.

Chapter 15 Cooking Techniques

PROJECT Culinary Review (continued)
Evaluate Food Browning

Step 2 Assess Food Browning

Directions Contrast each food item to assess how dry heat cooking affected the finished product. What happened to the color of each food item? What was the crust like? How did browning affect the flavor of each food item? Use the chart to record your observations about each food item's texture, flavor, and aroma.

Browning Results			
Food Item	Start Time	Stop Time	Observations

Name ______________________ Date ______________ Class ______________

Chapter 15 Cooking Techniques

PROJECT Culinary Review (continued)
Evaluate Food Browning

Step 3 Assess the Impact of Browning

Directions Using your observations from Step 2, answer the questions.

1. What did you observe about the start and stop times of the different food items you cooked? Explain your observations.

2. What differences did you notice between the different browned foods?

3. How could the observations you gathered about browning different food items impact customer opinions of a foodservice business?

For additional culinary projects and study tools, visit this book's Online Learning Center at **glencoe.com**.

Name ______________________ Date ____________ Class ____________

Chapter 16

Chapter 16 Seasonings and Flavorings

Section 16.1 Enhancing Food

Culinary Skills Project
Determine When to Season

Directions Read each of the cooking situations, and determine when to add the seasoning. Write your answer in the space provided.

1. **Food:** A large pot of chicken soup
   Seasoning: Salt
   When to add: ______________________________

2. **Food:** A beef roast
   Seasoning: Pepper
   When to add: ______________________________

3. **Food:** Baked stuffed pasta shells
   Seasoning: Red pepper
   When to add: ______________________________

4. **Food:** A custard sauce for a dessert
   Seasoning: Vanilla extract
   When to add: ______________________________

5. **Food:** Baked chicken
   Seasoning: Monosodium glutamate
   When to add: ______________________________

6. **Food:** Berber lamb stew
   Seasoning: Ground cinnamon
   When to add: ______________________________

7. **Food:** Tomato sauce
   Seasoning: Minced garlic
   When to add: ______________________________

Name ______________________ Date ______________ Class ____________

Chapter 16 Seasonings and Flavorings

Section 16.2 Herbs and Spices

Culinary Skills Project
Identify Herbs and Spices

Directions Smell the aroma of each of the herbs and spices in the numbered cups provided by your instructor. Identify each one by name and describe its key characteristics in the following chart.

Herb or Spice	Description
1.	
2.	
3.	
4.	
5.	
6.	
7.	
8.	
9.	

Name ______________________ Date ______________ Class ________

Chapter 16

Chapter 16 Seasonings and Flavorings

Section 16.3 Condiments, Nuts, and Seeds

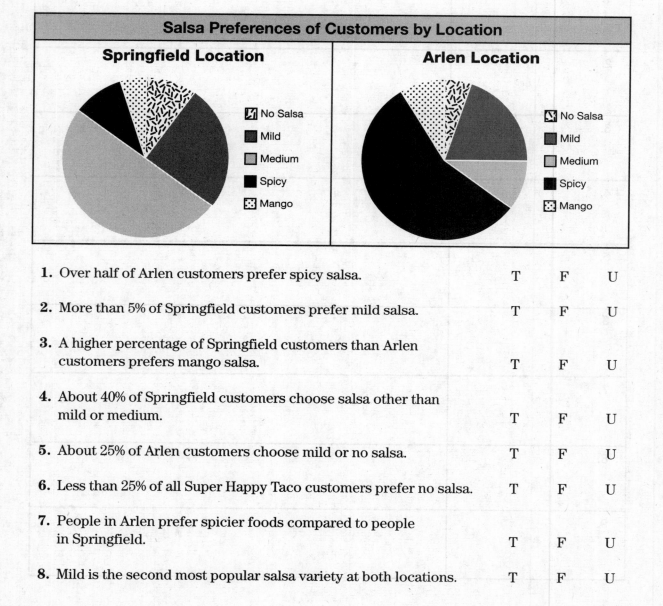

Mathematics Project
Compare Charts

NCTM Data Analysis and Probability Formulate questions that can be addressed with data and collect, organize, and display relevant data to answer them.

Directions Super Happy Taco is a quick-service restaurant with two different locations. The charts below display the salsa preferences for customers at each location. Study the charts, then circle whether each statement below is true (T), false (F), or unknown (U; if the answer cannot be found by looking at the charts).

Salsa Preferences of Customers by Location

1. Over half of Arlen customers prefer spicy salsa.	T	F	U
2. More than 5% of Springfield customers prefer mild salsa.	T	F	U
3. A higher percentage of Springfield customers than Arlen customers prefers mango salsa.	T	F	U
4. About 40% of Springfield customers choose salsa other than mild or medium.	T	F	U
5. About 25% of Arlen customers choose mild or no salsa.	T	F	U
6. Less than 25% of all Super Happy Taco customers prefer no salsa.	T	F	U
7. People in Arlen prefer spicier foods compared to people in Springfield.	T	F	U
8. Mild is the second most popular salsa variety at both locations.	T	F	U

Name ______________________ Date ______________ Class ________

Chapter 16 Seasonings and Flavorings

Section 16.4 Sensory Perception

NCTE 4 Use written language to communicate effectively.

English Language Arts Project

Evaluate Sensory Appeal

Directions Read the descriptions of different meals. Based on information from Section 16.4 in your textbook, evaluate whether the meal would be appealing, and explain why or why not.

Meal 1: Baked chicken breast, mashed potatoes with a white cream sauce, steamed cauliflower

Evaluation: ______________________________

Meal 2: Pasta with tomato sauce, sprinkled with grated Parmesan cheese, served with a green salad with tomatoes

Evaluation: ______________________________

Meal 3: Braised pork chop with caramelized onions, steamed green beans with almonds, and pilaf-style rice

Evaluation: ______________________________

Meal 4: Tuna casserole and creamed corn

Evaluation: ______________________________

Name ____________ Date ________ Class ________

Chapter 16 Seasonings and Flavorings

Study Skills
Using Note Cards

Directions Read the tips for using note cards to organize research. Then, imagine you will write a paper about seasonings and flavorings in food. Using Chapter 16 as a resource, fill in the sample note cards.

Tips for Using Note Cards
Sometimes, you have to do research to write a paper or give a presentation. You can organize your research using note cards that you fill in with information on the subject you are studying. • In the upper left corner, write the topic of your research. • In the upper right corner, write the name of the source. • In the body of the card, enter a single fact, quote, or thought that you would like to include in your paper or presentation. • Organize your cards to mirror the outline of your paper. • Keep a separate set of cards for each type of resource you have used, such as books, magazines, or films.

TOPIC: SOURCE:

Fact:

TOPIC: SOURCE:

Fact:

TOPIC: SOURCE:

Fact:

Name ______________________ Date ______________ Class ____________

Chapter 16 Seasonings and Flavorings

Certification Test Practice

Evaluating Test Results

Directions Read the following tips for evaluating test results, then answer the questions.

How to Evaluate Test Results
When you get a graded test back, you have the opportunity to reflect on what you have learned, what you have not learned, and your overall performance. Begin by looking at your mistakes. Find out the correct answers to the items you missed. Summarize in writing the material you had trouble with. You have the power to improve your performance on the next test!

1. What is the difference between a seasoning and a flavoring?

2. How does monosodium glutamate enhance food?

3. How would you use green peppercorns?

4. Why should whole spices be added to food early in the cooking process?

5. How should fresh nuts and seeds be stored?

Chapter 16

Name ______________________ Date ____________ Class ________

Chapter 16 Seasonings and Flavorings

Content and Academic Vocabulary
English Language Arts

NCTE 12 Use language to accomplish individual purposes.

Directions Correctly use 10 of the vocabulary terms in a short essay.

Content Vocabulary		Academic Vocabulary
seasoning	condiment	distinct
flavor enhancer	seed	opaque
flavoring	nut	complement
spice	sensory properties	indication
herb	savory	
bouquet garni	plate composition	

Name ______________________ Date ____________ Class __________

Chapter 16 Seasonings and Flavorings

PROJECT Culinary Review
Taste-Test Seasonings

Scenario Seasonings and flavorings, herbs and spices, and condiments can enhance and even change the flavor of the foods to which they are added. In this project, you will boil potatoes, add various seasonings and flavorings to them, and describe their flavors.

Academic Skills You Will Use	Culinary Skills You Will Use
ENGLISH LANGUAGE ARTS **NCTE 5** Use different writing process elements to communicate effectively. **SCIENCE** **NSES 1** Develop an understanding of science unifying concepts and processes: evidence, models, and explanation.	• Moist cooking techniques • Seasoning foods • Sensory evaluation

Step 1 Boil Your Potatoes

Directions Follow your teacher's instructions to form small groups. As a group, peel, cube, and boil four medium potatoes. Follow all safety and sanitation precautions as you cook. Separate the potatoes into seven small batches. Taste the first batch of potato without any seasoning or flavoring added, and describe its flavor.

Batch #1: Plain potatoes (no seasoning)

Name ______________________ Date ______________ Class ______________

Chapter 16

Chapter 16 Seasonings and Flavorings

PROJECT Culinary Review (continued)
Taste-Test Seasonings

Step 2 Add Seasonings and Flavorings

Directions Choose two different seasonings and flavorings for each category, and mix with the other batches of potatoes.

Seasonings and Flavorings
Add a different seasoning or flavoring to two batches of potatoes. Make your selection using the information from Section 16.1 of your textbook. Write your selections in the chart.

Batch #2		Batch #3	
Seasoning/Flavoring Used		Seasoning/Flavoring Used	
Amount Used		Amount Used	

Herbs and Spices
Add a different herb or spice to two batches of potatoes. Make your selection using the information from Section 16.2 of your textbook. Write your selections in the chart.

Batch #4		Batch #5	
Herb/Spice Used		Herb/Spice Used	
Amount Used		Amount Used	

Condiments
Add a different condiment to two batches of potatoes. Make your selection using the information from Section 16.3 of your textbook. Write your selections in the chart.

Batch #6		Batch #7	
Condiment Used		Condiment Used	
Amount Used		Amount Used	

Name ______________________ Date ____________ Class ________

Chapter 16 Seasonings and Flavorings

PROJECT **Culinary Review** (continued)
Taste-Test Seasonings

Step 3 Describe the Flavors

Directions Taste each seasoned batch of potatoes. Describe the flavor in the chart. Compare it with the flavor of the unseasoned batch you tasted. Use creative language in your descriptions.

Flavor Comparisons	
Batch	**Flavor Description**
Batch #2	
Batch #3	
Batch #4	
Batch #5	
Batch #6	
Batch #7	

For additional culinary projects and study tools, visit this book's Online Learning Center at **glencoe.com.**

Name ______________________ Date ____________ Class ________

Chapter 17 Breakfast Cookery

Section 17.1 Meat and Egg Preparation

Culinary Skills Project
List Breakfast Food Cooking Techniques

Directions Write the cooking procedure for each breakfast food listed in these charts. Use Section 17.1 in your textbook as a guide.

Ham	
Step 1	
Step 2	

Bacon (Done in the Oven)	
Step 1	
Step 2	
Step 3	
Step 4	
Step 5	

Shirred Eggs	
Step 1	
Step 2	
Step 3	
Step 4	
Step 5	
Step 6	

Chapter 17

Name ______________________ Date ______________ Class __________

Chapter 17 Breakfast Cookery

Section 17.2 Breakfast Breads and Cereals

NCSS I E Culture Demonstrate the value of cultural diversity, as well as cohesion, within and across groups.

Social Studies Project

Research the Pancake

Directions Use at least two different sources, including books, magazines, cookbooks, and the Internet, to research the history of the pancake. Then, answer the questions.

1. What cultures feature pancakes as part of their cuisine?

____

____

____

____

2. How do pancakes rise?

____

____

____

____

3. What kinds of toppings can be used with pancakes?

____

____

____

____

4. How can pancakes be used in meals?

____

____

____

____

____

____

Chapter 17

Name ______________________ Date ______________ Class __________

Chapter 17 Breakfast Cookery

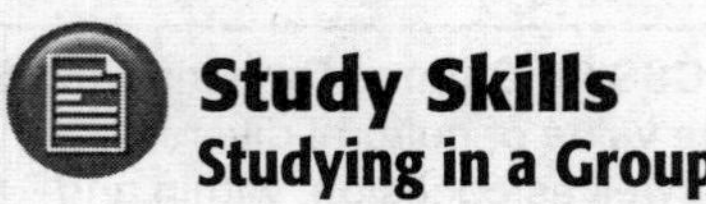

Study Skills
Studying in a Group

Directions Read the tips for successful group study. Then, write a paragraph about group study using each of the academic vocabulary words from Chapter 17.

Study Successfully in a Group
• Ask two or three others to come with you. • Select a leader. The leader's task is to develop an agenda that can keep everyone in the group focused on studying. • Before the group meets, the leader assigns sections of the text to each member. Members should read the entire text, and then write questions covering their assigned section. • Schedule enough time for your group to cover all the material. Make sure there is time for questions and discussion. • During the session, take turns asking and answering one another's questions. • All members of the group should come to the session prepared to answer questions. This will help everyone be prepared for an upcoming class discussion, project, or test. • Plan for a short social time before and after the session. Take at least one short break during the session. The leader should keep track of time and get everyone focused after a break.

designate	mainstay
alternative	function

____

____

____

____

____

____

____

____

____

____

Name ______________________ Date ____________ Class __________

Chapter 17 Breakfast Cookery

Certification Test Practice
Jogging Your Memory

Directions Read the tips for jogging your memory. Then, take the multiple-choice test. Circle the letter of the correct answer to each question.

Tips to Jog Your Memory
Sometimes you know the answer, but you cannot remember it during the test. Try these techniques to help you jog your memory: • Relax and slowly reread the question. • Put a mark next to the question, and then go on to the next question. • Recall material that relates to the question, and then revisit the question. • Try writing the question on the back of your test. Writing can jog your memory.

Chapter 17

1. Fresh eggs are better for poaching because
a. older eggs taste funny when poached.
b. older eggs will fall apart in the poaching liquid.
c. older eggs will have a flatter yolk when poached.
d. older eggs will turn a slightly gray color when poached.

2. For the best results, eggs used for frying should be
a. Grade AA.
b. Grade A.
c. Grade B.
d. Grade C.

3. A quick-service breakfast should include
a. eggs, bacon, toast, and coffee.
b. hash browns, pancakes, and fruit.
c. French toast, ham, and yogurt.
d. Any of the above.

4. Granular cereals include
a. grits, barley, and farina.
b. oatmeal and cracked wheat.
c. boxed sugar-coated loops.
d. popcorn.

Name ______________________ Date ____________ Class ________

Chapter 17 Breakfast Cookery

Content and Academic Vocabulary
English Language Arts

NCTE 12 Use language to accomplish individual purposes.

Directions Circle the letter of the phrase that best completes the sentence.

1. **Albumin** is
   - **a.** a portfolio for pictures.
   - **b.** the shell that protects an egg.
   - **c.** where most of an egg's calories can be found.
   - **d.** the thickest part of the white that surrounds the yolk of an egg.

2. **To curdle** means to
   - **a.** coagulate.
   - **b.** separate.
   - **c.** bind together.
   - **d.** digest.

3. **Shirred** refers to
   - **a.** eggs baked with cream and bread crumbs.
   - **b.** pleats in a dress.
   - **c.** beaten eggs.
   - **d.** a flan.

4. If an egg is **porous**, it means.
   - **a.** it is easily poured
   - **b.** it is easily broken.
   - **c.** flavors and odors can be absorbed through the shell.
   - **d.** it is rotten.

5. When you choose a **side order**, you
   - **a.** get an order of food in addition to the main dish.
   - **b.** get the special of the day.
   - **c.** get an entrée.
   - **d.** get a double order of food.

6. An **omelet** is
   - **a.** an egg dish made of beaten eggs cooked without stirring.
   - **b.** exactly the same as a frittata.
   - **c.** eggs baked with cream and bread crumbs.
   - **d.** another name for fried eggs.

7. A **soufflé** is
   - **a.** an egg dish made of whole eggs.
   - **b.** another name for quiche.
   - **c.** a breakfast meat.
   - **d.** a puffed egg dish baked in the oven.

Chapter 17

Name ______________________ Date ______________ Class __________

Chapter 17 Breakfast Cookery

PROJECT

Culinary Review

Produce Breakfast Orders

Scenario Timing is very important when producing orders for breakfast. Some breakfast foods are cooked very quickly, while others take more time. In this project, you will review several breakfast orders, decide which foods must be cooked first, and produce several breakfast orders at one time.

Academic Skills You Will Use	Culinary Skills You Will Use
SCIENCE **NSES F** Develop an understanding of personal and community health. **MATHEMATICS** **NCTE Measurement** Apply appropriate techniques, tools, and formulas to determine measurements.	• Sanitation and safety knowledge • Dry cooking techniques • Production timing

Chapter 17

Step 1 Review Breakfast Orders

Directions Follow your teacher's directions to form groups. Review the breakfast orders as a group. List the ingredients you will need for each order.

Breakfast Order #1	Breakfast Order #2	Breakfast Order #3
Pancakes with a side of bacon	Two fried eggs over easy with a side of white toast	Oatmeal with a side of sliced fruit

Ingredients needed: ____

Name ______________________ Date ______________ Class __________

Chapter 17 Breakfast Cookery

PROJECT Culinary Review (continued)
Produce Breakfast Orders

Step 2 Make a Production Schedule

Directions Determine the order in which the breakfast foods must be cooked for all orders to be ready at the same time. List the information in the chart.

Breakfast Production Schedule	
Task	**Time for Task**

Chapter 17

Name ______________________ Date ____________ Class ________

Chapter 17 Breakfast Cookery

PROJECT Culinary Review (continued)
Produce Breakfast Orders

Step 3 Serve Breakfast

Directions If possible, make the breakfast orders, or a variation supplied by your teacher. Then, answer the questions.

1. What was the easiest part of making the three breakfast orders?

____

____

____

____

2. What was the most difficult part of making the three breakfast orders?

____

____

____

____

3. What skills do you think line cooks need to be able to handle cooking breakfasts to order?

____

____

____

____

4. What role does the service staff play in a successful breakfast service?

____

____

____

____

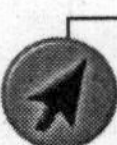

For additional culinary projects and study tools, visit this book's Online Learning Center at glencoe.com.

Name ______________________ Date ____________ Class ________

Chapter 18 Garde Manger Basics

Section 18.1 What Is Garde Manger?

Culinary Skills Project
Create a Flower Garnish

Directions Create a lily flower garnish using the following directions. Once you have finished, have your teacher evaluate it, and answer the questions.

How to Create a Lily Garnish
1. Gather the following supplies: turnips, beets or rutabagas at least 3 inches in diameter, a carrot, or lemon, a mandoline, a paring knife or zester, and wooden toothpicks. **2.** Wash and trim the ends of the vegetables. **3.** Make paper-thin slices of the vegetables (except the carrot or lemon) using the mandoline. **4.** Cut julienne strips of the carrot, or cut several strips of lemon zest to form the center of the lily. **5.** Roll the first vegetable slice tightly around a strip of carrot or lemon zest to form a petal. Hold at the base. **6.** While tightly holding the base of the lily center, loosely wrap the bottom of another vegetable slice around the base of the lily, opposite the previous slice. **7.** Continue wrapping 3 to 5 vegetable slices around the lily. Fasten at the base using toothpicks. **8.** Chill in ice water until the lily petals are firm.

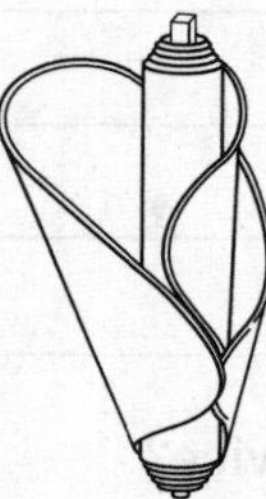

Step 5: Rolling the center of the lily

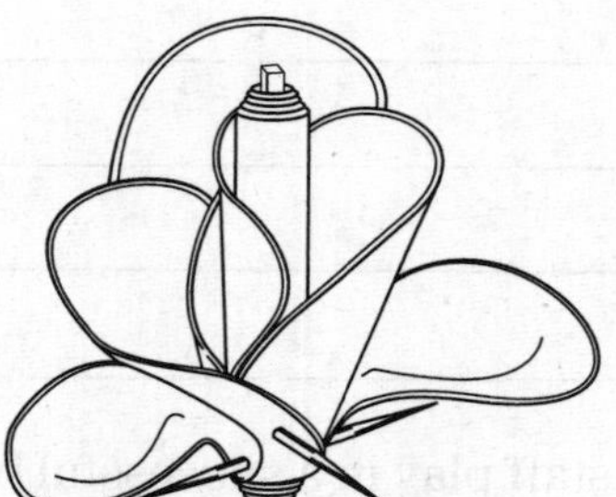

Step 7: Making lily petals

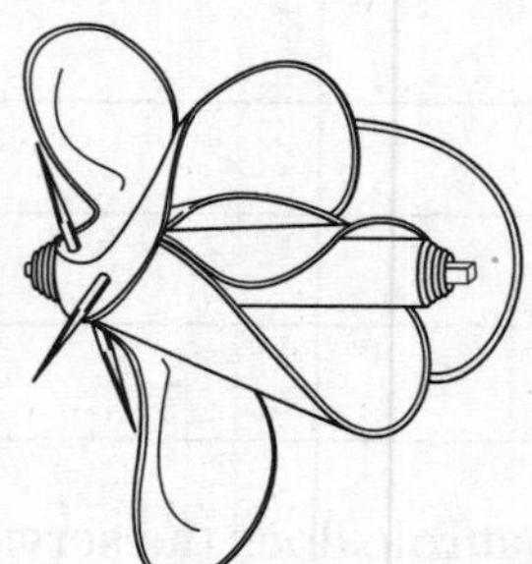

Step 8: The finished lily

1. How easy or difficult were the vegetable slices to work with?

____

____

2. What might you have done differently to make the garnish easier to work with?

____

____

Chapter 18

Name ______________________ Date ______________ Class ____________

Chapter 18 Garde Manger Basics

Section 18.2 Salads and Salad Dressings

NCTM Number and Operations
Compute fluently and make reasonable estimates.

Mathematics Project
Cost Food Waste for a Fruit Salad

Directions These fruit salad ingredients have less than a 100% edible portion yield. Use these formulas to find your answers:

Quantity ÷ Edible Portion % = As Purchased (AP)
As Purchased (AP) − Quantity = Waste/Trim
Waste/Trim × Unit Cost = Waste/Trim Cost

Quantity	Ingredient	Edible Portion %	As Purchased (AP)	Waste/ Trim	Unit Cost	Waste/ Trim Cost
1½ lbs.	Pineapple, cubed	52%			$2.50/lb.	
3 lbs.	Orange sections	70%			$0.58/lb.	
2 lbs.	Cantaloupe, cubed	54%			$0.87/lb.	
4 lbs.	Strawberries, sliced	76%			$2.59/lb.	
½ lb.	Apples, sliced	76%			$0.85/lb.	
5 oz.	Raspberries, whole	97%			$0.33/oz.	
3½ lbs.	Grapefruit sections	47%			$0.45/lb.	
¾ lb.	Bananas, sliced	68%			$0.65/lb.	
2½ lbs.	Grapes, whole	83%			$2.99/lb.	
1¾ lbs.	Nectarines, sliced	86%			$1.49/lb.	
			Total Cost of Trim Loss			

Chapter 18

Name ______________________ Date ____________ Class __________

Chapter 18 Garde Manger Basics

Section 18.3 Cheese

NCTE 3 Apply strategies to interpret texts.

English Language Arts Project

Describe Cheese Use in Recipes

Directions Choose a recipe that uses cheese as one of its main ingredients. Once you have chosen a recipe, attach a copy of the recipe to this page, and answer the questions.

1. What type(s) of cheese does your recipe use?

____

____

2. Describe the type(s) of cheese your recipe uses.

____

____

____

____

3. How is the cheese used in your recipe?

____

____

____

____

____

4. Are there other types of cheeses that could be used in your recipe? Explain which cheeses might be good substitutes.

____

____

____

____

____

____

Chapter 18

Name ______________________ Date ______________ Class __________

Chapter 18 Garde Manger Basics

Section 18.4 Cold Platters

Culinary Skills Project
Diagram a Fruit Platter

Directions Use colored pencils or markers to diagram the layout of a fruit platter. Label each piece of fruit and its position on the platter, and identify any garnishes you decide to use. Take into account the colors and textures of the different types of fruit you would use when you plan where they will go on the platter.

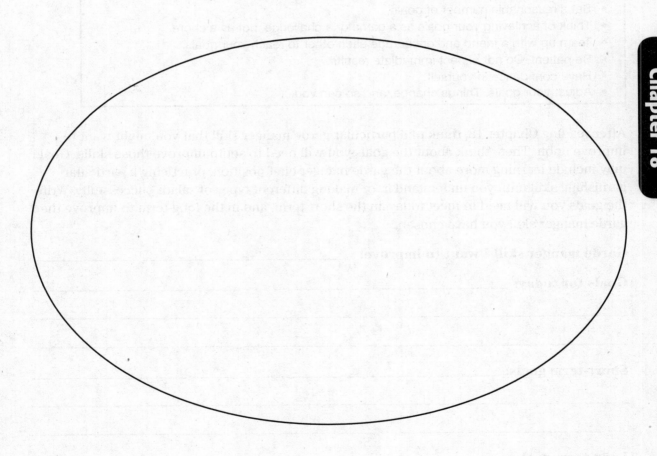

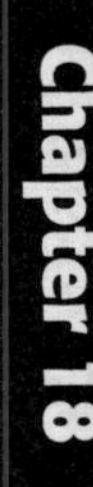

Name ______________________ Date ____________ Class ________

Chapter 18 Garde Manger Basics

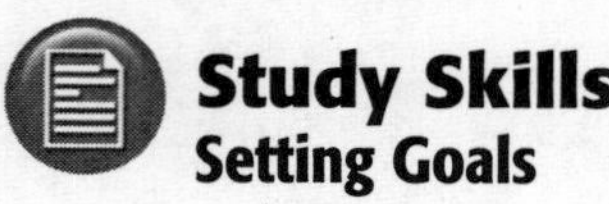

Study Skills
Setting Goals

Directions Read the tips for setting goals for success. Then, follow the prompt to write educational goals for today, the short-term, and the long-term that can help you sharpen your garde manger skills.

Tips to Set Goals for Success
Good students set realistic goals to help them achieve success. They create a plan for success and then work to make that plan a reality. • Make your goals clear, specific, and measurable. • Make sure your goals are realistic. • Phrase your goals positively. • Set a reasonable number of goals. • Think of achieving your goals as a game or a challenge, not as a chore. • Team up with a friend and encourage each other to reach your goals. • Be patient. Do not expect immediate results. • Have confidence in yourself. • Adjust your goals. Things change, and so can you.

After reading Chapter 18, think of a particular garde manger skill that you might want to improve upon. Then, think about the goals you will need to set to improve those skills. Goals may include learning more about the garde manger chef position, practicing a particular garnishing skill until you understand it, or making different types of salads successfully. Write the goals you will need to meet today, in the short-term, and in the long-term to improve the garde manger skill you have chosen.

Garde manger skill I want to improve: ______________________

Goals for today: ______________________

____

____

Short-term goals: ______________________

____

____

Long-term goals: ______________________

____

____

Name ______________________ Date ______________ Class ______________

Chapter 18 Garde Manger Basics

Certification Test Practice

Scanning for Information

Directions Read the tips on how to scan text. Then, scan the section on Flavor-Adding Greens on page 465 of your textbook to answer the questions.

How to Scan Text for Information
Scanning is a reading technique that can help you find information within a text quickly. If your teacher gives you a study guide with words or concepts that will appear on an upcoming test, you can use scanning to locate them in your text and review them. Scanning is also helpful during an open book test. • Use a key word or phrase contained in the questions. • Let your eyes move quickly over the material, looking only for the key word or phrase. • Your mind will likely pick up more than you think you are seeing. Stop scanning when you see the key word or phrase. • Read the paragraph around the key word or phrase to understand its meaning and the way the word will be used.

________ **1.** How are these leaves classified?

________ **2.** What greens have leaves that look like dandelion leaves?

________ **3.** What do these greens add to salads?

________ **4.** What greens have long and spiky leaves?

________ **5.** What type of green grows in running streams?

________ **6.** What type of green is commonly known as a weed that grows in a lawn?

________ **7.** Which greens have short creamy white or pale yellow leaves?

________ **8.** What greens that are commonly cooked are sometimes added to salads?

________ **9.** The leaves of this salad green look like spinach leaves, but have a slight lemony taste.

________ **10.** Two different greens have curly leaves. Which are they?

Chapter 18

Name ______________________ Date ______________ Class ____________

Chapter 18 Garde Manger Basics

Content and Academic Vocabulary
English Language Arts

NCTE 12 Use language to accomplish individual purposes.

Directions In the space provided, write the vocabulary term or terms that correctly completes the sentence. The first one is done for you. You will not use all the terms.

Content Vocabulary		Academic Vocabulary
canapé	cheddaring	appropriate
garde manger brigade	ripening	subtle
charcuterie	emulsifier	beneficial
tournée	finger food	whet
salad	crudité	
vinaigrette	relish tray	

1. Jonelle liked to serve a(n) ___appropriate___ accompaniment to her braised veal entrée.

2. Xavier prepared ______________ of jicama, carrots, and celery for the awards dinner.

3. The ______________ Noel made contained balsamic vinegar mixed with olive oil.

4. The school's dietitian added a(n) ______________ of walnuts, apples, and lettuce to the lunch menu.

5. The ______________ of cold meats and cheeses served at the local Italian restaurant is meant to ______________ the appetite.

6. Adding Greek olives, pickled cauliflower, and other colorful marinated vegetables to the ______________ showed Allie's creativity.

7. ______________, consisting of stuffed mushrooms, tartlets, and tiny sausages, was served at the art exhibit.

8. The mold in cheese is actually ______________ because it gives it a unique flavor.

9. Often, herbs are added to cheese, which give it a(n) ______________ flavor.

10. The ______________ consists of employees who each specialize in a particular type of cold food preparation.

Chapter 18

Name ______________________ Date ____________ Class ________

Chapter 18 Garde Manger Basics

PROJECT Culinary Review
Build a Salad

Scenario Salads can be interesting additions to a meal, or even a meal themselves. They can be easily customized. In this project, you will choose a salad type, research local and seasonal ingredients that can be added, and make the salad.

Academic Skills You Will Use	Culinary Skills You Will Use
SOCIAL STUDIES **NCSS I A Culture** Analyze and explain the ways groups, societies, and cultures address human needs and concerns **NCSS III E People, Places, and Environments** Describe, differentiate, and explain the relationships among various regional and global patterns of geographic phenomena, such as vegetation.	• Sanitation and safety knowledge • Garde manger skills • Salad preparation

Chapter 18

Step 1 Choose a Salad

Directions Follow your teacher's instructions to form small groups. As a group, select a type of salad. Then, answer the questions.

As a group, select one of the following types of salads:

- Appetizer salad
- Accompaniment salad
- Main-course salad
- Separate-course salad
- Dessert salad

Salad chosen: ______________________

1. Describe the type of salad you have chosen.

____

____

____

____

2. As a group, decide on the ingredients to use in your salad, and list them.

____

____

____

____

Name ______________________ Date ____________ Class ________

Chapter 18 Garde Manger Basics

PROJECT Culinary Review (continued)
Build a Salad

Step 2 Research Local/Seasonal Ingredients

Directions Each group member should choose a local or seasonal ingredient that would enhance the salad you have planned. Write the ingredient you have chosen, and use this page to take notes about that ingredient. List your sources.

Local/Seasonal Ingredient: ______________________________

Notes: ______________________________

Chapter 18

Name ______________________ Date ____________ Class ________

Chapter 18 Garde Manger Basics

PROJECT Culinary Review (continued)
Build a Salad

Step 3 Make Your Salad

Directions If possible, make your salad as a group, including at least one of the local/seasonal ingredients chosen. If you have made the salad, taste it. Answer the questions.

1. What other menu items would go with your salad?

2. What effect do you think the chosen ingredient has on the salad?

3. How would you market your salad with the local/seasonal ingredient?

4. Why do you think it is important to add local/seasonal ingredients to standard dishes?

For additional culinary projects and study tools, visit this book's Online Learning Center at glencoe.com.

Chapter 18

Name ______________________ Date ____________ Class ____________

Chapter 19 Sandwiches and Appetizers

Section 19.1 Sandwich-Making Basics

Culinary Skills Project
Create Nutritious Sandwiches

Directions Review the information on MyPyramid food groups from Chapter 11 in your textbook, and online at **www.mypyramid.gov**. Use the information to create three sandwich options that use items from all of the food groups. List the ingredients in each sandwich, as well as the food groups to which they belong.

Sandwich #1 ____

____

____

____

____

____

____

Sandwich #2 ____

____

____

____

____

____

____

Sandwich #3 ____

____

____

____

____

____

____

Chapter 19

Name ______________________ Date ____________ Class ____________

Chapter 19 Sandwiches and Appetizers

Section 19.2 Sandwiches

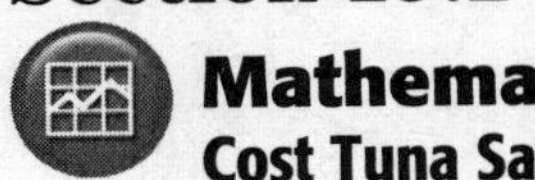

Mathematics Project
Cost Tuna Salad Ingredients

NCTM Number and Operations
Understand the meanings of operations and how they relate to one another.

Directions Use the form to calculate the total cost, the cost per serving, and the selling price for tuna salad. Divide the Unit Cost price by Unit Cost amount to get the price per unit. Then, multiply that amount by the Amount Needed to get the Extended Cost.

Recipe: Tuna Salad
Recipe Yield: 10
Cost per Serving:
Total Cost:

Ingredient	Amount Needed	Unit Cost	Extended Cost	Mark-Up = 25%
Tuna Fish	24 oz.	66 oz./$5.39		Calculate mark-up **(Total Cost × Mark-up)**
Sweet Relish	½ c.	$0.95/c.		
Mayonnaise	1 c.	$0.31/c.		
Salt	1 tsp.	$0.03/tsp.		Calculate total selling price **(Total Cost + Mark-Up)**
Eggs	2	$0.06 each		
Celery, Diced	½ c.	$0.25/c.		
Onion, Diced	2 Tbsp.	$0.03/Tbsp.		Calculate cost per serving **(Total Cost ÷ Recipe Yield)**
Pineapple Tidbits	8 oz.	$0.58/16 oz.		

Name ______________________ Date ______________ Class ______________

Chapter 19 Sandwiches and Appetizers

Section 19.3 Hot Appetizers

Culinary Skills Project

Describe Appetizer Service Types

Directions Describe the three styles of appetizer service listed. Then, choose an appetizer service style for each situation.

Appetizer Service Styles

Table Service ____

____

____

____

Buffet Service ____

____

____

____

Butler Service ____

____

____

____

1. ______________________ A party in an outdoor garden, with limited seating
2. ______________________ A wedding reception at a banquet hall
3. ______________________ A Sunday brunch buffet
4. ______________________ A cocktail party in an informal atmosphere
5. ______________________ A birthday dinner at a fine-dining restaurant
6. ______________________ A cocktail party in a formal atmosphere
7. ______________________ A dinner for two in a casual-dining restaurant

Name ______________________ Date ______________ Class ____________

Chapter 19 Sandwiches and Appetizers

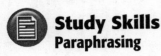

Study Skills
Paraphrasing

Directions Read the tips for paraphrasing text. Then, read the paragraphs from Chapter 19 and paraphrase them on the lines provided.

Tips for Paraphrasing Text

Paraphrasing is restating ideas in your own words. It helps you learn to take notes as you read. Paraphrasing also helps you to focus on the main idea and not get bogged down by details. When you paraphrase a reading passage, you do the following:

- Use your own words to express the main ideas from a piece of spoken or written communication.
- Distinguish between main ideas and less-important details, and focus on the main ideas.
- In your notes, use words and phrases instead of sentences.

1. Plate hot sandwiches on hot plates, and cold sandwiches on cold plates. Garnish the plates as appropriate for the type of sandwich. Many sandwiches are cut in half diagonally to show the fillings and to create a dramatic presentation. Frilled toothpicks are often used to keep sandwich halves from falling apart.

____

____

____

____

____

2. Presentation is key in serving appetizers. If appetizers are served buffet-style, arrange them so that they seem to flow toward guests. If plated, use plates and trays with interesting shapes and sizes. Notice how the appetizers look on the plate. Do not pack them in. Be sure to leave some open space on the plate. Add a small garnish for presentation.

____

____

____

____

____

Name ____________________ Date ____________ Class ____________

Chapter 19 Sandwiches and Appetizers

Certification Test Practice
Improving Your Attitude

Directions Read the tips for improving your attitude. Then, take the fill-in-the-blank test. Fill in the blanks using vocabulary terms from Chapter 19. Three of the vocabulary terms will not be used. Write them, along with their definitions, at the bottom of the page.

Tips to Improve Your Attitude
Attitude plays a big role in determining how well you study for and perform on tests. To keep a positive attitude: • Believe that what you are studying has long-term benefits for your life. • Be patient with yourself and know that learning takes time. • Think about the rewards you can give yourself if you meet your goals. • Remember that you have the power to develop and change. If you do poorly on a test today, you have the opportunity to do better next time.

croissant	emphasize	mayonnaise
pita	Monte Cristo	proportional
tortilla	foundation	maintain

1. The right garnish can ________ the fresh ingredients in a sandwich.
2. A(n) ________ sandwich has bread that is dipped in egg batter and then fried or grilled.
3. The perfect ________ for any sandwich is fresh bread.
4. A round-shaped flat bread that can be cut open to form a pocket is called a(n) ________.
5. The top and bottom slices of bread for a sandwich should be ________ for the sandwich to be easy to pick up.
6. A flaky ________ can make a good addition to a breakfast or as a roll for a sandwich.

Write the vocabulary words and their definitions that were not used above:

7. ____________________
8. ____________________
9. ____________________

Chapter 19

Name ______________________ Date ____________ Class ________

Chapter 19 Sandwiches and Appetizers

Content and Academic Vocabulary
English Language Arts

NCTE 12 Use language to accomplish individual purposes.

Directions Read the vocabulary term in the first column of the chart. Write what you think the term means in the second column. Use your textbook to learn the definition of the term and write it in the third column. If the definition in the text matches your prediction, put a check in the third column.

Terms	Predict What They Mean	Write the Dictionary Definition
variation		
au jus		
crêpe		
bouchée		
club sandwich		
obtain		
barquette		
Pullman loaf		
phyllo		
croissant		
focaccia		

Chapter 19

Name ______________________ Date ____________ Class ________

Chapter 19 Sandwiches and Appetizers

PROJECT Culinary Review
Organize Sandwich Making

Scenario Sandwiches often must be made in large quantities. This takes organization and planning skills. In this project, you will form groups and decide on a sandwich type, create a diagram of your workspace, and write production guidelines for making your sandwich in quantity.

Academic Skills You Will Use	Culinary Skills You Will Use
ENGLISH LANGUAGE ARTS **NCTE 5** Use different writing process elements to communicate effectively. **NCTE 12** Use language to accomplish individual purposes.	• Sanitation and safety knowledge • Making food in large quantities • Sandwich making

Step 1 Choose a Sandwich Type

Directions Follow your teacher's instructions to form groups. Decide on a type of sandwich to make; you may be assigned your sandwich type by your teacher.

Hot Sandwich	Cold Sandwich
Grilled Sandwich	Pizza Sandwich

Determine the ingredients your group will need to make your sandwich, including any garnishes and accompaniments, and the tools you will need to make the sandwich. Record your answers in the chart.

Sandwich Ingredients and Tools	
Category	**Selections**
Sandwich Type	
Bread	
Spread	
Filling	
Cheese	
Garnish	
Accompaniment(s)	
Tools	

Chapter 19

Name ____________________ Date __________ Class __________

Chapter 19 Sandwiches and Appetizers

PROJECT Culinary Review (continued)
Organize Sandwich Making

Step 2 Create a Workspace Diagram

Directions Imagine that your group will make 10 of the sandwiches you have chosen. Decide which group members will perform each part of the sandwich-making process. Use the space given to draw a diagram of where each group member will be placed in the workspace.

Task Assignments	
Name	**Task**

Chapter 19

Name ______________________ Date ____________ Class ____________

Chapter 19 Sandwiches and Appetizers

PROJECT Culinary Review (continued)
Organize Sandwich Making

Step 3 Write Production Guidelines

Directions Write guidelines for each group member to follow as he or she performs the assigned task. The guidelines should be easy to understand and use direct, clear language. If possible, once your guide is complete, make the sandwiches to test your organization skills.

Group Member #1 ______________________________

____

____

____

Group Member #2 ______________________________

____

____

____

Group Member #3 ______________________________

____

____

____

Group Member #4 ______________________________

____

____

____

Group Member #5 ______________________________

____

____

____

For additional culinary projects and study tools, visit this book's Online Learning Center at glencoe.com.

Chapter 19

Name ______________________ Date ____________ Class __________

Chapter 20 Stocks, Sauces, and Soups

Section 20.1 Stocks

Culinary Skills Project
Compare Stocks

Directions Follow your teacher's instructions to form groups. As a group, heat a homemade basic stock, or create one from scratch using information in Section 20.1 of your textbook. Then, make a corresponding commercial base stock. Taste the two stocks, fill out the ingredient lists, and answer the question.

Basic Stock

Name: ____

Ingredients: ____

____

Cooking Process: ____

____

____

Commercial Stock

Name: ____

Ingredients: ____

____

Cooking Process: ____

____

____

What differences did you notice between the two completed stocks?

____

____

____

____

____

____

Name ______________________ Date ____________ Class ____________

Chapter 20 Stocks, Sauces, and Soups

Section 20.2 Sauces

Science Project

Compare a Roux and a Reduction

NSES B Develop an understanding of interactions of energy and matter.

Directions Follow your teacher's instructions to form teams. Work as a team to create two sauces, using recipes from your teacher: one that you will thicken with a roux, and one that you will thicken by reduction. What were the differences in your methods and your results? What were the differences, if any, between the sauces? Write a report of your findings.

Roux vs. Reduction

Chapter 20

Name ______________________ Date ______________ Class __________

Chapter 20 Stocks, Sauces, and Soups

Section 20.3 Soups

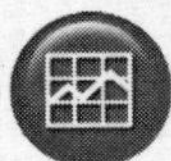

Mathematics Project
Calculate Soup Portions

NCTM Algebra Understand patterns, relations, and functions.

Directions Soupy's Restaurant sells seafood chowder in 6-ounce cup portions and 12-ounce bowl portions. On Monday, Soupy's Restaurant sold a total of 144 ounces of seafood chowder. Use this information to answer the questions.

1. Write an algebraic equation representing the amount of each size of seafood chowder that Soupy's sold on Monday, with x representing the quantity of cups and y representing the number of bowls.

____

2. Rearrange the equation you wrote in Question 1 so that y is isolated to one side (the equation should begin "$y =$").

____

3. Using the equation in Question 2, solve for y for each of the values given for x:

Values of Variables

x	0	2	4	6	8	10	12	14	16	18	20	22	24
y													

4. Using the values for x and y in Question 3, draw a graph of the equation in Question 2. (Plot each pair of x, y values, then connect the points with a line)

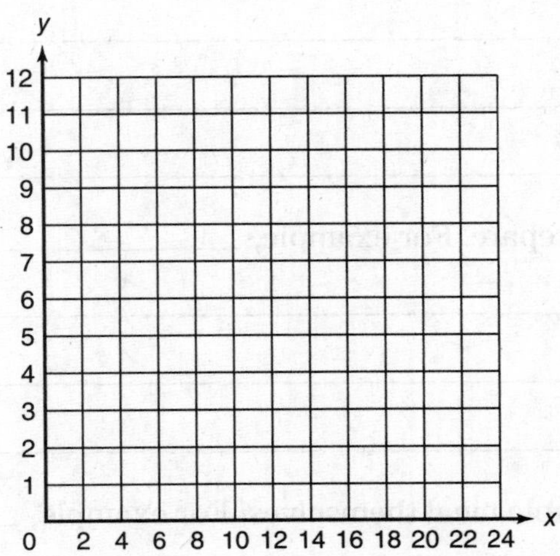

Chapter 20

Name ______________________ Date ______________ Class ____________

Chapter 20 Stocks, Sauces, and Soups

Study Skills
Giving Examples

Directions Read the tips for giving examples. Then, in your own words, write an example to support the statements from Chapter 20. One example is completed for you.

How to Give Examples
Examples help you convey your message and make your communication more interesting and valid. Tips for giving examples include: • Any time you express a main idea, think of examples that will support it. • The easiest place to find examples is real life. If you write, "Many recipes use a stock as part of their ingredients," you can think of recipes you know and use them as examples to support your statement. • When you make a verbal statement during a class discussion, have at least two examples prepared to support it. • Organize your writing and speech to have examples after your main point.

1. Stocks can be used in many different recipes. For example, a beef stew might use beef stock as a main ingredient, to give the stew a rich flavor.

2. It can take a lot of time to make a good sauce. For example, ______________________

3. Roux can be tricky to prepare. For example, ______________________

4. Some soups can be a whole meal themselves. For example, ______________________

Chapter 20

Name ______________________ Date ____________ Class ________

Chapter 20 Stocks, Sauces, and Soups

Certification Test Practice
Motivating Yourself

Directions Read the tips for motivating yourself for tests. Then, write one paragraph to answer each of the questions.

Tips to Motivate Yourself for Tests
• List as many reasons as you can think of to want to study and pass the test. • Spend a few minutes visualizing yourself studying thoroughly and earning an A on the test. Note how you feel when you imagine seeing the A grade. • Make a list of goals you want to achieve in your future. Consider how succeeding in school now can influence your ability to meet those goals. • Visualize your reward for doing well on the test. A reward may be a sense of accomplishment, making your parents proud, or raising your grade point average.

1. Why is studying for and passing tests important?

____

____

____

____

____

2. How can succeeding in school help you to reach your goals for the future?

____

____

____

____

____

3. What reward would you choose for doing well on a test?

____

____

____

____

____

Name ____________________ Date ____________ Class ________

Chapter 20 Stocks, Sauces, and Soups

Content and Academic Vocabulary

English Language Arts

NCTE 12 Use language to accomplish individual purposes.

Directions Use each vocabulary term to write one sentence that shows that you understand the term's meaning. The first one is completed for you.

1. supplement Winona thought she might **supplement** her homemade soup with a can of beef broth.
2. sauce ____________________
3. roux ____________________
4. bisque ____________________
5. fumet ____________________
6. characteristic ____________________
7. chowder ____________________
8. base ____________________
9. raft ____________________
10. mother sauces ____________________
11. mirepoix ____________________

Chapter 20

Name ______________________ Date ____________ Class __________

Chapter 20 Stocks, Sauces, and Soups

PROJECT Culinary Review
Create a Mother Sauce

Scenario The five mother sauces can be a base for many other types of sauces, called compound sauces. In this project, you will choose and describe a mother sauce, research a compound sauce, and make both sauces.

Academic Skills You Will Use	Culinary Skills You Will Use
ENGLISH LANGUAGE ARTS **NCTE 1** Read to understand texts. **NCTE 6** Adjust language to communicate effectively.	• Sanitation and safety knowledge • Moist cooking techniques • Seasoning and flavoring • Following recipes

Step 1 Choose a Mother Sauce

Directions Follow your teacher's instructions to form groups. As a group, choose one of the five mother sauces:

- Espagnole/demi-glace
- Tomato
- Velouté
- Béchamel
- Hollandaise

Describe the sauce you have chosen.

Sauce: ________________________________

Description: ________________________________

____

____

____

____

____

____

____

____

____

____

____

____

Name ______________________ Date ______________ Class ____________

Chapter 20 Stocks, Sauces, and Soups

PROJECT Culinary Review (continued)
Create a Mother Sauce

Step 2 Research a Compound Sauce

Directions Use Internet and print resources to find a compound sauce recipe that uses the mother sauce your group has chosen. Copy the recipe here, and write a short essay about its origins and uses.

____

____

____

____

____

____

____

____

____

____

____

____

____

____

____

____

____

____

____

____

____

____

Name ______________________ Date ______________ Class ______________

Chapter 20 Stocks, Sauces, and Soups

PROJECT Culinary Review (continued)
Create a Mother Sauce

Step 3 Make the Sauces

Directions As a group, choose one compound recipe. Make the mother sauce and the compound sauce you have chosen. Once you have finished, taste each sauce. Then, answer the questions.

1. What were the challenges you found in making the mother sauce?

2. What were the challenges you found in making the compound sauce?

3. What were the differences in flavor between the two sauces?

4. Why might a chef choose to make a compound sauce?

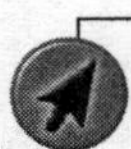

For additional culinary projects and study tools, visit this book's Online Learning Center at glencoe.com.

Name ______________________ Date ____________ Class ____________

Chapter 21

Chapter 21 Fish and Shellfish

Section 21.1 Fish Basics

Social Studies Project

Research a Fish Dish

> **NCSS I E Culture** Demonstrate the value of cultural diversity, as well as cohesion, within and across groups.

Directions Use Internet and print resources to find a dish from another culture that uses fish as one of its main ingredients. Attach a copy of the recipe to this sheet. Then, answer the questions.

Recipe Chosen: ______________________________

1. What are the origins of this dish?

____
____
____
____
____

2. How is the fish cooked in the dish?

____
____
____
____
____

3. What seasonings and spices are used in the dish?

____
____
____
____

4. Are there variations of the dish?

____
____
____
____

Name ______________ Date __________ Class __________

Chapter 21 Fish and Shellfish

Section 21.2 Shellfish Basics

Culinary Skills Project

Select Fish and Shellfish

Chapter 21

Directions Read each situation in the chart. Determine whether you should select the piece of fish or shellfish described. Then, explain why or why not in the right column.

Fish/Shellfish Purchasing Scenarios	
Situation	**Your Response**
The whole fish are slimy	
The crabs are warm and have a strange odor	
The meat of the flounder does not separate when the fillet is bent	
The raw shrimp in the shell is brown in color	
The clams are sandy on the inside	
The ocean bass smells like seaweed	
The gills on the flounder are pink	
The eyes of the catfish are sunken	
Ice is inside the frozen trout	
The lobsters are alive and brown in color	

Name ______________ Date ______________ Class ______________

Chapter 21 Fish and Shellfish

Section 21.3 Cooking Fish and Shellfish

Mathematics Project

Cost Seafood

NCTM Number and Operations Compute fluently and make reasonable estimates.

Chapter 21

Directions Complete the following math problems. Show your calculations in the space provided.

1. A seafood vendor offers you a 20% discount off the total price if you purchase 25 gallons of shucked oysters. Each gallon sells for $70. If you bought 25 gallons of oysters, what would be your price without the discount? What would be your price with the discount?

2. A fish vendor offers salmon in two forms: drawn fish or skin-on fillets. The drawn fish sells for $3.95 per pound. After filleting a 9-pound fish, you determine that your trim loss is 35% per pound. The fillets sell for $5.25 per pound with a 5% trim loss per pound. Which form of salmon is the best value?

Name ______________________ Date ______________ Class ________

Chapter 21 Fish and Shellfish

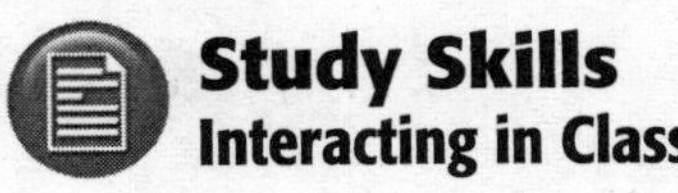

Study Skills
Interacting in Class

Directions Read the tips for interacting in class. Then, follow your teacher's instructions to form pairs. Read each question aloud and discuss it with your partner. Formulate an answer to each question based on the knowledge you have as a pair.

Tips to Interact in Class
• Use good listening skills. • Do your homework so you are prepared to respond to others. • Review your notes from the previous day and read ahead in your textbook. • Answer questions that the teacher raises. • Ask questions about the material being discussed. • Make contributions to small group discussions and projects.

1. What are the three different categories of fish, and their characteristics?

2. How should fresh fish be stored?

3. Describe two types of shellfish, and their characteristics.

4. What is surimi, and how is it used?

Name ______________________ Date ______________ Class __________

Chapter 21 Fish and Shellfish

Certification Test Practice

Using the Four Rs

Directions Read the tips for using the four Rs of test taking—read, recite, repeat, relax—to learn information that you will need to know on a test. Then, take the true/false test. Write a **T** for true or an **F** for false on the line beside the question.

Using the Four Rs for Tests

The following four Rs can help you better retain information that you will need to know on a test:

- *Read* the material on which you will be tested.
- *Recite* the important points aloud.
- *Repeat* the first two steps until you know the material.
- *Relax* on the day of the test. If you are tense, it will be hard to remember material.

These techniques may help you remember the correct answer:

- If you have trouble remembering the answer to a question, relax, close your eyes, take a deep breath, and visualize the text that you read.
- Next, in your mind, listen to yourself reciting the material.

1. ______ Fish are naturally tender because they have little connective tissue.

2. ______ Butterflied filets resemble an open book.

3. ______ Fresh fish is not usually graded, so the person receiving it must inspect it carefully.

4. ______ Type 2 USDC inspection for fish and shellfish covers processing methods and the processing plant.

5. ______ Live oysters that do not move when tapped should be thrown away.

6. ______ When purchasing shrimp, the smaller the shrimp, the lower the count.

7. ______ Crayfish are available year-round.

8. ______ Fatty fish are not as likely to dry out during cooking as lean fish.

9. ______ Baked fish should reach an internal temperature of 145°F (63°C) or above for 15 seconds.

10. ______ Whole fish and fish steaks that are thicker than 1½ inches are the best choices for broiling.

Name ______________________________ Date ______________ Class __________

Chapter 21 Fish and Shellfish

Content and Academic Vocabulary
English Language Arts

NCTE 12 Use language to accomplish individual purposes.

Chapter 21

Directions Choose the vocabulary term from the list that best completes each sentence. Write the word in the right column of the table. The first one is completed for you. You will not use all of the words.

Content Vocabulary		Academic Vocabulary	
flat fish	univalve	classify	mandatory
round fish	bivalve	keep	sufficient
drawn	cephalopod		
freezer burn	crustacean		
drip loss	flake		
mollusk	en papillote		

Definition	Example	Word
sufficient	The whole fish entrée was ______ for serving four people.	enough
The loss of moisture that occurs as fish thaws	It is best to cook small pieces of fish while still frozen to lessen ________.	
Food wrapped in parchment paper and cooked with vegetables, herbs, and sauces	The recipe for Risa's halibut called for the fish to be steamed ______.	
A shellfish that has no internal skeletal structure	An oyster is a ______ one classification of shellfish known as a _________.	
To break away in small layers	It is best to use moist-heat cooking for fish so that the flesh will ______ easily.	
Discoloration and dehydration caused by moisture loss as a food freezes	Wrap fish well in plastic before freezing to help prevent _________.	
Required	Inspection for accurate labeling, safety, and wholesomeness of frozen and canned fish is _______.	
A shellfish with a single shell	A conch is an example of a ___________.	
Fish that have had their gills and entrails removed	When Erik went to the fish market, he purchased a whole fish already _________.	

Name ____________________ Date ____________ Class ____________

Chapter 21 Fish and Shellfish

Chapter 21

PROJECT Culinary Review
Create Shrimp Dishes

Scenario Seafood can be used to create a variety of dishes. In this project, you will describe proper storage procedures for fresh shellfish, research different recipes, and answer questions about those recipes.

Academic Skills You Will Use	Culinary Skills You Will Use
ENGLISH LANGUAGE ARTS **NCTE 12** Use language to accomplish individual purposes. **SCIENCE** **NSES F** Develop an understanding of personal and community health.	• Sanitation and safety knowledge • Storage techniques • Recipe knowledge

Step 1 Describe Proper Storage

Directions Imagine that you work at a restaurant. You receive an extra shipment of fresh shrimp. In the space provided, describe how you would store the shrimp for later use.

How to store fresh shrimp:

Name ______________________ Date ____________ Class ________

Chapter 21 Fish and Shellfish

PROJECT Culinary Review (continued)
Create Shrimp Dishes

Step 2 Choose Shrimp Recipes

Directions Use Internet and print resources to find three different shrimp recipes. List the ingredients of each recipe, and describe how the shrimp is used in each.

Recipe #1: ______________________________

Ingredients: ______________________________

____

____

Use of Shrimp: ______________________________

____

____

Recipe #2: ______________________________

Ingredients: ______________________________

____

____

Use of Shrimp: ______________________________

____

____

Recipe #3: ______________________________

Ingredients: ______________________________

____

____

Use of Shrimp: ______________________________

____

____

Name ______________________ Date ______________ Class ________

Chapter 21 Fish and Shellfish

PROJECT Culinary Review (continued)
Create Shrimp Dishes

Step 3 Choose a Recipe to Make

Directions Choose one of the recipes from Step 2, and answer the questions. If possible, make the recipe you have chosen.

1. How would you describe your chosen recipe on a menu?

____

____

____

____

____

2. For what part of a meal would your chosen recipe be best? What type of restaurant might serve your chosen recipe?

____

____

____

____

____

3. Could a substitution be made for the shrimp in your recipe?

____

____

____

____

4. Why might a chef want to make a substitution for shrimp in a recipe?

____

____

____

____

For additional culinary projects and study tools, visit this book's Online Learning Center at glencoe.com.

Name ______________________ Date ______________ Class ____________

Chapter 22 Poultry Cookery

Section 22.1 Poultry Basics

NSES C Develop an understanding of the behavior of organisms.

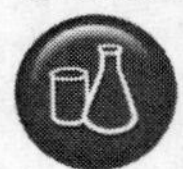

Science Project

Identify Poultry Characteristics

Directions List the physical characteristics and habitat for each kind of poultry.

Chicken ____

____

____

____

Turkey ____

____

____

____

Goose ____

____

____

____

Duck ____

____

____

____

Pigeon ____

____

____

____

Guinea ____

____

____

____

Chapter 22

Name ______________________ Date ______________ Class ________

Chapter 22 Poultry Cookery

Section 22.2 Cooking Poultry

Culinary Skills Project
Compare Poultry Textures

Directions Follow your teacher's instructions to form teams. As a team, cook three small pieces of chicken in three different ways:

- Sautéing
- Pan-Frying
- Baking

Once the chicken is completely done, taste each piece of chicken and answer the questions.

1. Describe any taste differences between the three pieces of chicken.

____

____

____

____

____

____

2. Describe any texture differences between the three pieces of chicken.

____

____

____

____

____

____

3. Describe any appearance differences between the three pieces of chicken.

____

____

____

____

____

____

Chapter 22

Name ______________________ Date ______________ Class ________

Chapter 22 Poultry Cookery

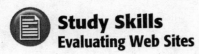

Study Skills
Evaluating Web Sites

Directions Read the tips for evaluating Web sites. Then, apply the tips as you use the Internet to research how poultry is raised. Identify and research how one kind of poultry is raised for human consumption. Write a paragraph about your findings.

How to Evaluate Web Sites
Before using a Web site for research, ask these questions to help you evaluate the site: • Are the writers authorities on the subject that you are researching? If so, what are their credentials? • Is the site timely? When was it created? When was it last updated? • Do the writers cite other Web sites or authorities? If so, are they legitimate? • Is this a local, state, national, or foreign government site? • Is this a Web site for an educational institution, such as a college or university?

Poultry-Raising Methods

Chapter 22

Name ______________________ Date ______________ Class ________

Chapter 22 Poultry Cookery

Certification Test Practice
Taking Online Tests

Directions Read the tips for taking online tests. Then, take the multiple-choice test. Fill in the bubble of the correct answer.

Tips for Taking Online Tests
Before the online test, ask your teacher these questions: • Will I see one question at a time, or can I scroll through the entire exam? • Will the questions be text only, or will there be illustrations? • Will I need to answer each question before I can go on to the next question? • Can I skip difficult questions and return to them later? • Can I review the test once I am done? • How do I change an answer?

Chapter 22

1. The term maturity refers to a poultry's
   - ○ age.
   - ○ sex.
   - ○ size.
   - ○ height.

2. Poultry that has been prepared and packaged for use is called
   - ○ ready-to-use.
   - ○ ready-to-cook.
   - ○ partially prepared.
   - ○ service-ready.

3. Poultry that has received a Grade A should have all the following characteristics except
   - ○ plump and meaty.
   - ○ clean skin.
   - ○ pinfeathers.
   - ○ intact bones.

4. The term roasting in poultry cookery is usually used when cooking
   - ○ turkeys.
   - ○ whole birds.
   - ○ chicken legs.
   - ○ ducks or geese.

5. ____________ are ideal for broiling or grilling.
   - ○ Large birds
   - ○ Giblets
   - ○ Trussed chickens
   - ○ Poultry pieces

6. There should never be more than one layer of chicken in a frying basket because
   - ○ the pieces will stick together.
   - ○ the chicken will not cook.
   - ○ the oil will cool.
   - ○ the batter coating will be too crispy.

7. Simmering is a cooking technique usually used for
   - ○ older, tougher birds.
   - ○ younger, tender birds.
   - ○ game birds.
   - ○ whole birds.

Name ______________________ Date ______________ Class __________

Chapter 22 Poultry Cookery

Content and Academic Vocabulary

English Language Arts

NCTE 12 Use language to accomplish individual purposes.

Directions Write the vocabulary term that best completes each sentence. You will not use all of the terms. The first one is done for you. You will not use all of the terms.

Content Vocabulary		Academic Vocabulary	
poultry	render	acceptable	indicate
kind	baste	process	principle
connective tissue	dredging		
giblets	stuffing		
market form	cavity		
trussing	ready-to-cook (RTC)		

1. Chris waited for the thermometer to reach 165°F to indicate that the roasted chicken was done.

2. Birds that get more exercise will have more ______________.

3. Jan knew that ______________ the turkey with twine would allow for an attractive final product.

4. Remove the ______________, consisting of the liver, gizzard, and heart from the ______________ of the turkey before roasting.

5. The fat in the skin will ______________ when the poultry is cooked at a high temperature, resulting in a beautifully browned bird.

6. It is ______________ to serve pre-sliced poultry to customers in some restaurants, while other foodservice establishments prefer to carve tableside.

7. Tige preferred his grandmother's recipe for cornbread ______________ to accompany poultry.

8. The ______________ of ______________ includes coating poultry parts in seasoned flour.

9. The USDA categorizes poultry according to ______________, or species, such as geese, ducks, or pigeons.

10. Sheryl's mom taught her to ______________ her chicken with its own juices as it roasts in the oven.

Chapter 22

Name ______________________ Date ____________ Class ____________

Chapter 22 Poultry Cookery

PROJECT Culinary Review
Create a Simmered Poultry Dish

Scenario Simmered poultry also creates a flavorful liquid that can be used in many types of sauces. In this project, you will cut poultry into pieces, simmer it, create a sauce, and evaluate your results.

Academic Skills You Will Use	Culinary Skills You Will Use
ENGLISH LANGUAGE ARTS **NCTE 12** Use language to accomplish individual purposes. **SCIENCE** **NSES B** Develop an understanding of interactions of energy and matter.	• Sanitation and safety knowledge • Moist cooking techniques • Making sauces

Chapter 22

Step 1 Cut Up Poultry

Directions Follow your teacher's instructions to form groups. Inspect the bird provided by your instructor. In the space provided, record the kind and type of poultry, and its age. Then, describe the quality characteristics of your bird. Once you are finished, cut the bird into pieces as described on pages 572–573 of your textbook.

Poultry Kind and Type: ______________________

Poultry Age: ______________________

Quality Characteristics: ______________________

____

____

____

____

____

____

____

____

____

Name ______________________ Date ____________ Class __________

Chapter 22 Poultry Cookery

PROJECT Culinary Review (continued)
Create a Simmered Poultry Dish

Step 2 Simmer Your Poultry

Directions As a group, select a recipe for simmering poultry that includes a sauce. Attach a copy of the recipe to this page. Prepare the poultry as directed in your recipe. Record the start time and end time for your cooking, and the internal temperature of the chicken, in the right column of the chart.

Simmering Poultry	
Recipe Name	
Start Time for Simmering	
End Time for Simmering	
Internal Temperature When Done	

Once the poultry is completely cooked, remove the poultry from the cooking liquid and prepare the sauce as directed in your recipe. After you are done, answer the questions.

1. What additional ingredients, seasonings, and/or flavorings did you use in your sauce?

____

____

____

____

2. How did you thicken your sauce? Describe any methods or ingredients you used.

____

____

____

____

3. How will your sauce complement the poultry you simmered?

____

____

____

____

Name ______________________ Date ______________ Class ______________

Chapter 22 Poultry Cookery

PROJECT Culinary Review (continued)
Create a Simmered Poultry Dish

Step 3 Evaluate Your Dish

Directions Taste your poultry to evaluate its appearance, flavor, and texture. Complete the evaluation.

Appearance: ______________________________

Flavor: ______________________________

Texture: ______________________________

For additional culinary projects and study tools, visit this book's Online Learning Center at glencoe.com.

Name ______________________ Date ______________ Class ________

Chapter 23 Meat Cookery

Section 23.1 Meat Basics

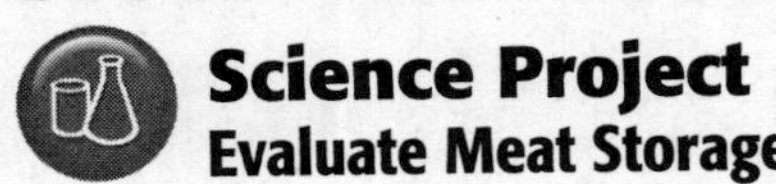

NSES F Develop an understanding of personal and community health.

Directions Read each situation and explain why the storage method is or is not appropriate. Write your answers on the lines provided.

1. **Fresh Chuck Roast** A chef at a casual-dining restaurant is preparing to order supplies for the week's menu. One of the dishes she plans to include is a chuck roast. If she buys the meat fresh on Tuesday and stores it in the refrigerator, what is the last day she can safely prepare the meat?

____

____

____

2. **Defrosted Pork Sausage** The line cook at a restaurant has defrosted pork sausage for Sunday brunch service. He keeps it safely stored in the refrigerator throughout the service, and has 8 pounds left over at the end of the day. How long can the defrosted meat stay safely in the refrigerator?

____

____

____

3. **Shelf Storage** A sous chef has just received a shipment from a beef vendor. She has decided to freeze half of the meat that was delivered. What is the best way to store the meat and avoid freezer burn?

____

____

____

4. **Seasoning Meat** A sous chef is helping to prepare the meat course of a wedding buffet. Some of his duties include defrosting and seasoning the prime rib before it is roasted. How long before putting the prime rib in the oven can the meat stay on the counter?

____

____

____

Chapter 23

Name ______________________ Date ______________ Class ____________

Chapter 23 Meat Cookery

Section 23.2 Meat Cuts

Culinary Skills Project
Identify Meat Cooking Methods

Directions In the chart, identify whether the fabricated cuts of meat listed are tender or not tender. Then, identify a cooking method for each fabricated cut. Label whether the cooking method is a moist, dry, or combination cooking method.

Pork		
Fabricated Cut	**Tender or Not Tender**	**Cooking Method**
Boston butt, boneless		
Spareribs		
Loin chops, center cut		
Loin roast, boneless		
Fresh ham, skinned, short shank		
Loin, back ribs		

Lamb		
Fabricated Cut	**Tender or Not Tender**	**Cooking Method**
Shoulder, square cut, boneless		
Rib chops		
Loin chops		
Leg, boneless		
Foreshank		
Lamb for stewing		

Name ______________________ Date ____________ Class ________

Chapter 23 Meat Cookery

Section 23.3 Principles of Cooking Meat

English Language Arts Project

Evaluate a Meat Recipe

Directions Choose a meat recipe and attach a copy of the recipe to this page. Use the space provided to evaluate the ingredients, mise en place, equipment, and timing that will be needed to prepare this recipe.

Recipe Name: ______________________

Ingredients: ______________________

Mise en Place: ______________________

Equipment: ______________________

Timing: ______________________

Chapter 23

Name ____________________ Date ____________ Class ____________

Chapter 23 Meat Cookery

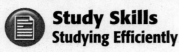

Study Skills
Studying Efficiently

Directions Read the following tips on how to study efficiently. Then, apply the tips as you study an aspect of meat inspection and grading from Chapter 23.

How to Study Efficiently

- Select the appropriate time, environment, and place for studying.
- Focus on one section of text at a time.
- Mark any information you do not understand.
- After studying one section, stop and write down what you have learned in your own words.
- Go back to what you did not understand and reconsider the information.
- Consult your teacher if you still do not understand.

Read about meat in Chapter 23 (pages 586–613 of your textbook). Then, write about each topic in your own words, note the concepts you did not understand, and, if possible, clarify the confusing parts.

Chapter 23

Meat Inspection and Grading

How I understand it in my own words: The meat for foodservice operations must have a United States Department of Agriculture (USDA) Inspection Stamp.

What I do not understand: ____________________

Clarification of what I did not understand: ____________________

Name ______________________ Date ____________ Class ________

Chapter 23 Meat Cookery

Certification Test Practice
Improving Reading Comprehension

Directions Read the following tips for reading comprehension. Then, assess your reading comprehension by completing the sample test below.

Tips to Improve Reading Comprehension
To help your reading comprehension, ask yourself these questions while you read: • Do I understand the main point that the author is trying to make? • Can I identify the ways in which the author supports the main point? • Could I explain the author's message to someone else using my own words? • How does this relate to what I already know, or to my life?

Each statement listed is false. Rewrite each statement to make it true. You may have to delete words or phrases, add words or phrases, or make statements more specific.

1. Lamb shoulder is a fabricated cut of lamb that is often braised or roasted.

____

____

____

2. High-heat cooking is used on less-tender cuts of meat because it does not shrink the meat and helps break down the connective tissue to tenderize the meat.

____

____

____

3. Trichinosis is a virus that causes mild flu-like symptoms. The best way to avoid trichinosis is to properly refrigerate raw pork.

____

____

____

4. A marinade is a mixture of ground spices that is rubbed on raw food before it is cooked.

____

____

____

Chapter 23

Name ______________________ Date ____________ Class ________

Chapter 23 Meat Cookery

Content and Academic Vocabulary
English Language Arts

NCTE 12 Use language to accomplish individual purposes.

Directions Use each vocabulary term to write one sentence that shows you understand the term's meaning. The first one is completed for you.

1. meat

   The nutrients in **meat** include water, protein, and fat.

2. collagen

   ____

3. barding

   ____

4. marbling

   ____

5. yield grade

   ____

6. rest

   ____

7. primal cut

   ____

8. satisfy

   ____

9. elastin

   ____

10. composed

    ____

11. curing

    ____

Chapter 23

Name ______________________ Date ______________ Class ____________

Chapter 23 Meat Cookery

PROJECT

Culinary Review
Understand Meat Cuts

Scenario There are many meat cuts from which to choose. A chef must know the characteristics of each, and from where on the animal they come. In this project, you will identify primal and fabricated meat cuts, outline a carcass and primal cuts, and discuss differences and similarities between animals.

Academic Skills You Will Use	Culinary Skills You Will Use
SCIENCE **NSES C** Develop an understanding of matter, energy, and organization in living systems. **NSES C** Develop an understanding of biological evolution.	• Meat identification • Primal and fabricated cuts

Step 1 Identify Primal and Fabricated Cuts

Directions Review Chapter 23 of your textbook for the primal cuts of meat in the chart. Name some fabricated cuts for each primal cut listed.

Cuts of Meat	
Primal Cut	**Fabricated Cut**
Chuck	
Round	
Loin (near round and center cuts)	
Rib (rib loin)	
Brisket, Plate, Flank	

Chapter 23

Name ____________________ Date ____________ Class ____________

Chapter 23 Meat Cookery

PROJECT Culinary Review (continued)
Understand Meat Cuts

Step 2 Diagram Primal Cuts

Directions Choose one of the following types of meat: lamb, veal, or beef. In the space provided, draw an outline carcass of your chosen type of meat according to the illustrations on page 590 in your textbook. Divide the outline into the primal cuts (see page 598 for lamb; page 600 for veal; page 602 for beef). Label each primal cut correctly.

Name ______________________ Date ____________ Class __________

Chapter 23 Meat Cookery

PROJECT Culinary Review (continued)
Understand Meat Cuts

Step 3 Compare Information With Others

Directions As a class, compare charts. Discuss the similarities and differences, and then answer the questions.

1. How are the primal cuts similar to each other?

2. How are the primal cuts different from each other?

3. Look on page 596 of your textbook. Why do you think the primal cuts of pork are so different from the other types of meat?

For additional culinary projects and study tools, visit this book's Online Learning Center at glencoe.com.

Chapter 23

Name ______________________ Date ______________ Class ______________

Chapter 24 Pasta and Grains

Section 24.1 Pasta

Social Studies Project
Discover Asian Noodles

> **NCSS 1 A Culture** Analyze and explain the ways groups, societies, and cultures address human needs and concerns.

Directions Using print or Internet resources, research the following types of Asian noodles. Describe the characteristics of each noodle. Then, identify a dish and its country of origin for which each type of noodle could be used.

Asian Noodles		
Noodle Type	**Noodle Characteristics**	**Noodle Dish/ Country of Origin**
Clear Vermicelli		
Chinese Egg Noodles		
Egg Roll Skins		
Rice Noodles		
Rice Sticks		
Rice Papers		
Buckwheat Noodles		
Somen Noodles		
Cellophane Noodles		

Name ______________ Date ______________ Class ______________

Chapter 24 Pasta and Grains

Section 24.2 Rice and Other Grains

NSES A Develop abilities necessary to do scientific inquiry.

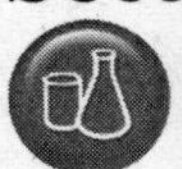

Science Project
Observe Absorption Rates

Directions Follow your teacher's instructions to form groups. As a group, cook three different samples of white rice:

1. Using 1 cup water and 1 cup rice
2. Using 2 cups water and 1 cup rice
3. Using 3 cups water and 1 cup rice

Simmer each rice sample on low heat for 15 minutes. Allow each sample to sit for 5 minutes, and check each sample. Then, answer the questions.

1. What happened to the rice in sample 1?

____

____

____

2. What happened to the rice in sample 2?

____

____

____

3. What happened to the rice in sample 3?

____

____

____

4. Why do you think the three rice samples turned out differently?

____

____

____

5. What can you determine about cooking grains from this experiment?

____

____

____

Chapter 24

Name ______________________ Date ____________ Class ________

Chapter 24 Pasta and Grains

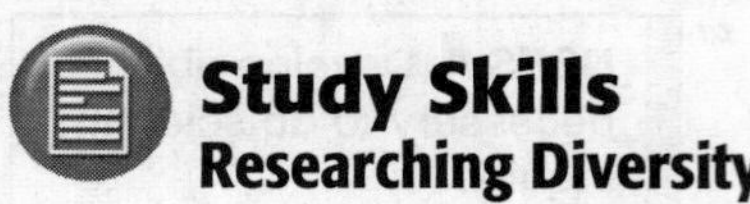

Study Skills
Researching Diversity

Directions Read the tips for researching diversity. Then, respond to the prompt to write eight questions you would ask to learn more about using pasta and grains in different ethnic cuisines.

Tips for Researching Diversity
Some school assignments ask you to research a different culture with which you may be unfamiliar. You may have to answer questions, write a paper, or give a presentation about another culture. When researching diversity, follow these tips: • Research such topics as special holidays, religious beliefs, traditions, language, music, art, food, style of dress, stories, myths, folk tales, and etiquette. • Use reading reference materials and appropriate Internet resources when researching other cultures. • Conduct interviews of people from different cultures to get a firsthand explanation of their culture. Prepare interview questions in advance. • Do not think only about how cultures are different from yours. Also consider the ways in which they are alike.

In Chapter 24, you read about the different types of pastas and grains, and how they are prepared and stored. Imagine that you are attending an ethnic food class for a culture with which you are not familiar. List questions you would ask the teacher during an information interview to understand more about the use of pasta and grains in the culture.

1. ______________________________

2. ______________________________

3. ______________________________

4. ______________________________

5. ______________________________

6. ______________________________

7. ______________________________

8. ______________________________

Chapter 24

Name ______________________ Date ____________ Class ________

Chapter 24 Pasta and Grains

Certification Test Practice
Using Self-Reflection

Directions Read the tips for self-reflection. Then, take the multiple-choice test shown. Fill in the bubble beside the term or phrase that does not relate to the concept in bold.

Tips for Self-Reflection
Self-reflection means to examine oneself. Understanding how your personality, your strengths, and your weaknesses influence the way you take tests can help you to improve. To encourage self-reflection, ask yourself these questions: • What has been my most stressful school-related experience? • How do I handle stress? • What tools do I use to manage my time? • What do I usually do to prepare for tests? • How do I feel in the hours and minutes leading up to a test? • How do I feel during a test? • In what ways might my personality influence my test-taking style? • What stress reduction and time management tools can I use to improve?

1. Rice
- ○ often served as part of a main dish
- ○ starchy seeds of a cereal grass
- ○ increases in volume as it cooks
- ○ must be soaked before cooking

2. Farfalle
- ○ can be boiled or baked
- ○ resemble bow ties
- ○ work well with medium or rich sauces
- ○ come from a seed grain

3. Serving pasta
- ○ often done alone on a plate with sauce
- ○ can wait until all other food items are cooked
- ○ is sometimes done on a soup plate
- ○ must be done when pasta is ready

4. Corn products
- ○ include polenta and hominy
- ○ can sometimes be eaten fresh
- ○ are not really grains
- ○ are sometimes served as a vegetable

5. Braising grains
- ○ creates fluffy grains that do not stick together
- ○ is a combination cooking method
- ○ is preferred to be done in the oven
- ○ requires no added oils or fats

6. Risotto method
- ○ food can be held for a while after cooking
- ○ continuous stirring is important
- ○ creates grains with a creamy consistency
- ○ seasonings can be added after sautéing

Chapter 24

Name ______________________ Date ____________ Class ________

Chapter 24 Pasta and Grains

Content and Academic Vocabulary

English Language Arts

NCTE 12 Use language to accomplish individual purposes.

Directions Write the letter of each vocabulary term on the line next to the definition. You will not use all the terms.

Content Vocabulary		Academic Vocabulary
a. pasta	g. wheat	m. labor
b. al dente	h. corn	n. achieve
c. grain	i. hominy	o. option
d. rice	j. masa harina	p. versatile
e. barley	k. pilaf method	
f. oat berry	l. risotto method	

______ **1.** To do; accomplish

______ **2.** A hardy, adaptable grain that can be grown in warm and cold climates

______ **3.** A finely ground hominy used in tortillas and breads

______ **4.** Grouts; a whole grain with texture and nutrients

______ **5.** Made by soaking dried corn in lye until kernels swell and outer layers loosen and can be removed

______ **6.** Braising involving sautéing the grain in oil or butter along with other ingredients before adding liquid

______ **7.** Grain is sautéed and then small amounts of hot liquid are added while stirring the grain

______ **8.** A starchy food product made from grains

______ **9.** Hard work

______ **10.** The starchy seeds of a cereal grass

______ **11.** "To the bite"; tender, yet firm

______ **12.** Adaptable

Chapter 24

Name ______________________________ Date ____________ Class __________

Chapter 24 Pasta and Grains

PROJECT Culinary Review
Cook and Stuff Pasta

Scenario Pasta should be cooked for a specific amount of time for it to turn out al dente, but not hard. In this project, you will cook three batches of pasta for differing amounts of time, describe the pastas' characteristics, and try stuffing each batch of pasta.

Academic Skills You Will Use	Culinary Skills You Will Use
ENGLISH LANGUAGE ARTS **NCTE 4** Use written language to communicate effectively. **SCIENCE** **NSES B** Develop an understanding of interactions of energy and matter.	• Sanitation and safety knowledge • Moist cooking methods • Determining doneness

Step 1 Cook Pasta

Directions Follow your teacher's instructions to form groups. Describe the boiling method of cooking pasta. Then, as a group, cook three small batches of manicotti, according to the times given in the chart.

Boiling Method of Cooking Pasta:

____

____

____

____

____

____

____

____

Manicotti Cooking Times	
Manicotti Batch	**Cooking Time**
Batch #1	5 minutes
Batch #2	10 minutes
Batch #3	20 minutes

Chapter 24

Name ______________________ Date ______________ Class ______________

Chapter 24 Pasta and Grains

PROJECT Culinary Review (continued)

Cook and Stuff Pasta

Step 2 Describe Cooked Pasta

Directions As each manicotti batch finishes, taste the pasta. Use the space provided to describe each batch's texture and flavor. Give explanations of why each batch tastes the way it does.

Batch #1: ______________________________

Batch #2: ______________________________

Batch #3: ______________________________

Chapter 24

Name ______________________ Date ____________ Class ____________

Chapter 24 Pasta and Grains

PROJECT Culinary Review (continued)

Cook and Stuff Pasta

Step 3 Stuff Pasta

Directions Use one manicotti noodle from each batch to stuff with a stuffing of your teacher's choice. After you have stuffed a manicotti noodle from each batch, answer the questions.

1. What were the differences in stuffing the three different manicotti batches?

2. What can you conclude about cooking pasta for a stuffed pasta dish?

3. What would you do with a batch of pasta for a stuffed pasta dish that had been overcooked?

4. Why is timing important in making pasta dishes?

For additional culinary projects and study tools, visit this book's Online Learning Center at **glencoe.com.**

Chapter 24

Name ______________ Date ______________ Class ______________

Chapter 25 Fruits, Vegetables, and Legumes

Section 25.1 Fruits

Science Project
Ripen Fruit

NSES B Develop an understanding of chemical reactions.

Directions Complete the following steps to ripen fruit. Answer the questions below.

1. Place one unripe apple, melon, or banana in a brown paper bag and seal it.
2. Observe the stages of ripening. Look for changes in color, firmness, and aroma. Check your fruit for changes after 24 hours. Record your results in the chart.
3. Check your fruit again after 48 hours, and again after 72 hours. Record your results in the chart.

Fruit	24 Hours	48 Hours	72 Hours

1. What happens to fruit when it ripens? ______________________________

2. Why will some fruits, such as apples, melons, and bananas, ripened in a sealed paper bag? ______________________________

3. How can you prevent fruit from becoming overripe? ______________________________

4. What are five fruits that do not ripen after harvest? ______________________________

Chapter 25

Name ______________________ Date ______________ Class __________

Chapter 25 Fruits, Vegetables, and Legumes

Section 25.2 Vegetables

Culinary Skills Project

Prepare Vegetables

Directions Select one of the following techniques. Then, prepare a work plan. List each step needed to perform the task. You may use the textbook and any information provided by your teacher. Practice your chosen technique several times. Then, prepare a demonstration and show the class how to properly perform your selected technique. Once you have given your presentation, answer the questions.

Julienne	Shocking
Blanching	Washing greens
Parboiling	Cutting vegetables on a mandoline

Technique chosen: ______________________

Work plan: ______________________

1. Describe the technique you have chosen. ______________________

2. What were the challenges in learning the technique? ______________________

3. What were the challenges in describing the technique to others? ______________________

Chapter 25

Name ______________________ Date ______________ Class ________

Chapter 25 Fruits, Vegetables, and Legumes

Section 25.3 Legumes

Mathematics Project

Count Beans

NCTM Algebra Use mathematical models to represent and understand quantitative relationships.

Directions Write and solve algebraic equations to answer the questions below.

1. A three-bean salad contains 1.5 times as many garbanzo beans as kidney beans, and 3 times as many kidney beans as green beans. If a bowl of three-bean salad contains 136 beans, how many of each type of bean are in the bowl?

2. Seth would like to make a two-bean salad with kidney beans (which have 15 grams of protein per cup) and green beans (2 grams of protein per cup). If he wants 2 cups of the finished salad to contain 20 grams of protein, how many cups of each type of bean should Seth use (rounded to the nearest ¼ cup)?

3. Last week, Eliza ordered two cases of canned kidney beans and three cases of canned green beans for a total order cost of $159. This week, she ordered one case of kidney beans and four cases of green beans for a total of $142. How much does each type of bean cost per case?

Name ______________________ Date ____________ Class ________

Chapter 25 Fruits, Vegetables, and Legumes

Study Skills
Improving Memorization Skills

Directions Read the tips for improving memorization skills. Then, write the correct fruit and vegetable family that best fits the description.

Tips to Improve Your Memorization Skills
• Think about what you are trying to learn. Find an interest in the material if you wish to memorize it with ease. • Study the items you wish to remember the longest. • Use concrete imagery whenever possible. Close your eyes and visualize the explanation and summary answer. Try to see it on the page.

	1. Has soft flesh, this skin, and one pit, or stone
	2. These come from flowering plants and contain at least one seed.
	3. These fruits ripen after they are picked and grow in hot climates. They are the best quality when they are firm, unblemished, plump, and have good color.
	4. These store and provide food to their plants. Those of good quality are firm and unwrinkled.
	5. Firm, thin-skinned fruit that grows on trees. They have a central core filled with tiny seeds. They may be harvested ripe, but they also ripen after they are picked.
	6. These fruits have a thick firm rind covered in a layer of colored skin, called the zest.
	7. These are often used for seasoning and flavoring because most have a strong taste and odor.
	8. These shrink when they are cooked because of their high water content.
	9. These grow on bushes and vines and are picked when they are fully ripened.
	10. These grow in clusters on vines. Their color and flavor is found mostly in their skin.
	11. Quality fruits are semisoft, slightly heavy, and have good color.
	12. These grow quickly in cool weather. They are served raw as well as cooked, and are firm and heavy for their size.
	13. This family of vegetables has large root systems and trailing vines. Their flowers are often edible in addition to the main vegetable.

Chapter 25

Name ______________________ Date ____________ Class ________

Chapter 25 Fruits, Vegetables, and Legumes

Certification Test Practice
Using Flashcards

Directions Read the tips for preparing for tests using flashcards. Then, use the chart to list the different types of beans. Use the completed chart to create your own flashcard study aids.

Prepare for Tests with Flashcards
• Keep up to date on reading the text and studying your notes. You will remember more of what you need to know for the test if you study a little each day. • Use flashcards for ideas and concepts that require shorter answers. • Keep your notes concise and easy to read. You will be able to review and scan them easily in the future if you stay organized.

Side A	Side B
	Flat shaped, pale green, with a smooth texture and sweet taste
	Medium-size, round, and beige colored; also called chick peas
	Larger than American white beans; they have a creamy color, mild flavor, and smooth texture
	Green or yellow in color; small, round, and with a floury texture
	Light brown, oblong kernels with a firm texture
	Small, white, and oval in shape; they have a powdery texture and mild flavor
	Medium-size, oval-shaped peas; they are beige in color with a black dot on the skin
	Creamy white, oval-shaped beans with a powdery texture and mild flavor
	Disk-shaped, pea-size beans; they are green or brown in color
	Large, flat, kidney-shaped beans; they are brown or white in color with a fine texture
	Reddish-brown, kidney-shaped beans

Name ______________________ Date ____________ Class ____________

Chapter 25 Fruits, Vegetables, and Legumes

Content and Academic Vocabulary
English Language Arts

NCTE 12 Use language to accomplish individual purposes.

Directions Correctly use 10 of the vocabulary terms in a short essay about a visit to a place that sells fruits and vegetables.

Content Vocabulary		Academic Vocabulary
drupe	net weight	diminish
ripe	packing medium	hasten
ethylene gas	mandoline	mark
compote	legume	accessible
chutney	pulse	
tuber	quick soak	

A Visit to a Fruit and Vegetable Market

Name ______________________ Date ______________ Class ________

Chapter 25 Fruits, Vegetables, and Legumes

PROJECT Culinary Review
Research Potatoes

Scenario Potatoes are a versatile ingredient for many types of cooking. Different potatoes have different uses, however, and you must know which to choose for an individual recipe. In this project, you will choose a potato, list its characteristics, preferred cooking methods, and growing information, and examine the potatoes firsthand.

Academic Skills You Will Use	Culinary Skills You Will Use
SCIENCE **NSES A** Develop abilities necessary to do scientific inquiry. **SOCIAL STUDIES** **NCSS III E People, Places, and Environments** Describe, differentiate, and explain the relationships among various regional and global patterns of geographic phenomena such as landforms, soils, climate, vegetation, natural resources, and population.	• Sanitation and safety knowledge • Vegetable identification • Ingredient use • Cooking method knowledge

Step 1 Choose a Potato Type

Directions Working individually, choose a variety of potato from the list. Describe the characteristics of the potato you choose in the space provided.

- Russet potato
- Red potato
- Yukon potato
- White sweet potato
- Red sweet potato
- Purple potato
- Fingerling potato

Potato type chosen: ________________________________

Potato characteristics: ________________________________

____

____

____

____

____

____

____

Name ______________________ Date ______________ Class ________

Chapter 25 Fruits, Vegetables, and Legumes

PROJECT Culinary Review (continued)
Research Potatoes

Step 2 Research Your Potato

Directions Use online and printed sources to research growing information about the potato type you chose. Look for information about its origins, where and how it is grown, and the length of time it can be stored. Use the space provided to take notes. Once you have gathered your information, share it with the rest of the class.

Chapter 25

Name ______________________ Date ______________ Class __________

Chapter 25 Fruits, Vegetables, and Legumes

PROJECT Culinary Review (continued)
Research Potatoes

Step 3 Identify Potatoes and Cooking Methods

Directions Follow your teacher's instructions to form groups. As a group, examine five varieties of potatoes provided by your teacher. Identify the type of potato, and assess its skin color and texture, and its interior color and texture. Record your observations in the chart.

Potato Type Observations				
Potato Type	Skin Color	Skin Texture	Interior Color	Interior Texture

As a group, determine whether each potato type you examined is mealy or waxy. Decide on appropriate cooking methods for each potato type. Record your answers in the chart.

Potato Type Observations		
Potato Type	Mealy or Waxy	Cooking Methods

For additional culinary projects and study tools, visit this book's Online Learning Center at **glencoe.com**.

Name ____________________ Date __________ Class __________

COMPETITIVE EVENTS PRACTICE

Make Chicken Chasseur

Directions Follow your teacher's instructions to form competition teams of two to four people. Each team will be given a recipe for chicken chasseur to make for competition. Special attention should be paid to safety and sanitation procedures.

Judging
In this competition, you will be judged on:
• How your team handles food safely • The appearance and flavor of your chicken chasseur • The sanitation procedures you follow • The cleanliness of your workspace

Preparation Phase

1. Write a work plan of how your team will make the chicken chasseur. Turn in a copy of your work plan to your teacher.

   ____

   ____

   ____

2. Prepare your workspace for competition. During preparation:
   - Retrieve all necessary equipment and tools
   - Observe all safety and sanitation procedures
   - Keep foods at the proper temperature
   - Use a sanitizing solution to clean your workspace before beginning

   Do not prepare any part of the chicken chasseur at this time.

Cooking Phase

1. Make your chicken chasseur, using the work plan you created. You must make two portions of your chicken chasseur—one to be tasted, and one for presentation. There should not be a visible difference between the two plates. You will have one hour to make your chicken chasseur.

2. Bring both plates to the tasting area designated by your teacher when it is completed and ready for judging, or at the end of the time period. Display your chicken chasseur with the work plan you wrote earlier.

Name ______________________ Date ______________ Class __________

COMPETITIVE EVENTS PRACTICE (continued)

Competitive Events Review

Once the competition has been completed, write a short essay on the experience of creating a more complex dish than the ones you have created for competition so far. How did you handle the extra ingredients? What were your biggest challenges? What would you have done differently next time?

Name ______________________ Date ______________ Class ______________

Chapter 26 Baking Techniques

Section 26.1 Bakeshop Formulas and Equipment

NCSS 1 Develop an understanding of science unifying concepts and processes: change, constancy, and measurement.

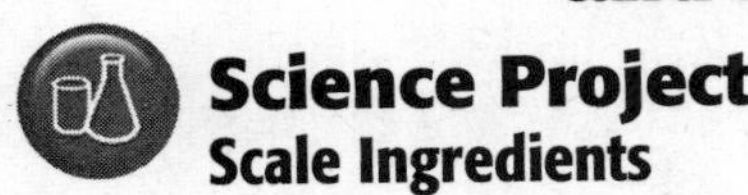

Science Project
Scale Ingredients

Chapter 26

Directions Scale the ingredients provided by your teacher by completing the steps. Then, answer the questions.

How to Scale Ingredients
1. Measure the flour, using a 1 cup volume measuring cup. 2. Weigh the flour on a balance or digital scale. 3. Record the weight in the chart. 4. Find the difference between the volume and the weight. Does the flour weigh 8 ounces? Record the weights in the chart. 5. Weigh the flour on a portion scale. Record the weight in the chart. 6. Repeat Steps 1–5 for each ingredient listed in the chart.

Ingredient Measuring and Weight

Ingredient Measured by Volume	Balance or Digital Scale Weight	Portion Scale Weight	Difference Between Volume and Weight
1 cup Flour			
1 cup Sugar			
1 cup Salt			

1. Was the weight by volume for each ingredient more or less than the balance or digital scale weight?

____

____

2. Was the portion scale weight for each ingredient different than the balance or digital scale weight?

____

____

3. What differences would you see in the finished product if you measured your ingredients by volume instead of weight?

____

____

Chapter 26 Baking Techniques

Section 26.2 Bakeshop Ingredients

Culinary Skills Project

Identify Bakeshop Ingredients

Directions Describe how each bakeshop ingredient listed in the chart is used in baking. Write your answers in the right column.

Bakeshop Ingredients	
Ingredient	**How It Is Used**
Bread Flour	
Cake Flour	
Pastry Flour	
Water	
Milk and Cream	
Vegetable Shortening	
Oil	
Granulated Sugar	
Eggs	
Baking Soda	
Yeast	
Salt	

Name ______________________ Date ____________ Class ____________

Chapter 26 Baking Techniques

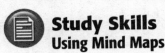

Study Skills
Using Mind Maps

Directions Read the steps for making a mind map. Then, select a passage from Chapter 26 to create a mind map that reflects your comprehension of the passage.

How to Make a Mind Map

Mind maps are a good way to organize related pieces of information and better comprehend your reading. In the center circle, write the main idea of the passage. In the outer circles, write details that support or explain the main idea. Use these steps:

1. Skim the passage and look for the most important idea.
2. Write a word or phrase about the main idea in the center circle.
3. Skim the passage again and look for concepts and details that support the main idea.
4. Write these concepts or details in the outer circles.
5. Carefully read the passage.
6. As you read, revise your mind map by adding clarity and details. Add more spokes and circles if necessary.

Baking Techniques

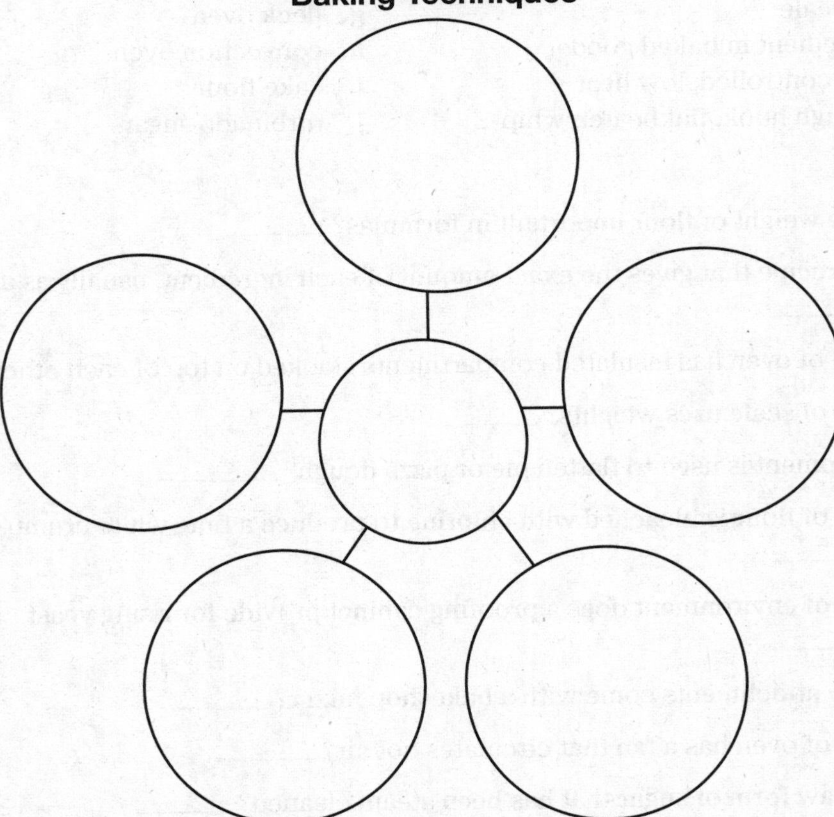

Name ____________ Date ____________ Class ____________

Chapter 26

Chapter 26 Baking Techniques

Certification Test Practice
Taking Open Book Tests

Directions Read the tips for preparing for open book tests. Then, open your text and use it to take the short answer test. Match the short answer to the question.

Tips to Prepare for Open Book Tests

- Keep up to date on reading the text and studying your notes. You may often use both the text and your notes in an open book test.
- If permitted, use sticky notes to mark certain points in your text that you feel are important. This will help you locate them quickly during a test.
- Mark your notes with a highlighter. This will help you to find the important points quickly during your test.
- Condense your notes into only those that are applicable to the test. Do not overburden yourself with too many notes. Time is limited when taking a test, so being prepared and organized is important.

Short Answers

a. formula
b. balance scale
c. core ingredient in baked goods
d. humidity controlled, low heat
e. spiral dough hook, flat beater, whip
f. sheeter
g. deck oven
h. convection oven
i. cake flour
j. turbinado sugar

Questions

1. Why is the weight of flour important in formulas? _______
2. What is a recipe that gives the exact amount of each ingredient, usually as a percentage, called? _______
3. What kind of oven has insulated compartments stacked on top of each other? _______
4. What type of scale uses weights? _______
5. What equipment is used to flatten pie or pizza dough? _______
6. What type of flour is bleached with chlorine to produce a fine, white crumb to baked goods? _______
7. What type of environment does a proofing cabinet provide for rising yeast dough? _______
8. What basic attachments come with a bakeshop mixer? _______
9. What kind of oven has a fan that circulates hot air? _______
10. What is a raw form of sugar that has been steam cleaned? _______

Name ______________________ Date ____________ Class __________

Chapter 26 Baking Techniques

Content and Academic Vocabulary

English Language Arts

NCTE 12 Use language to accomplish individual purposes.

Chapter 26

Directions Solve the crossword puzzle by answering the clues. You will not use all the vocabulary terms listed.

Content Vocabulary		Academic Vocabulary
scaling	staling	imprecise
stack oven	shortening	invaluable
springform pan	leavening agent	surround
sheet pan	yeast	contribution
gluten	fermentation	
crumb	dough	

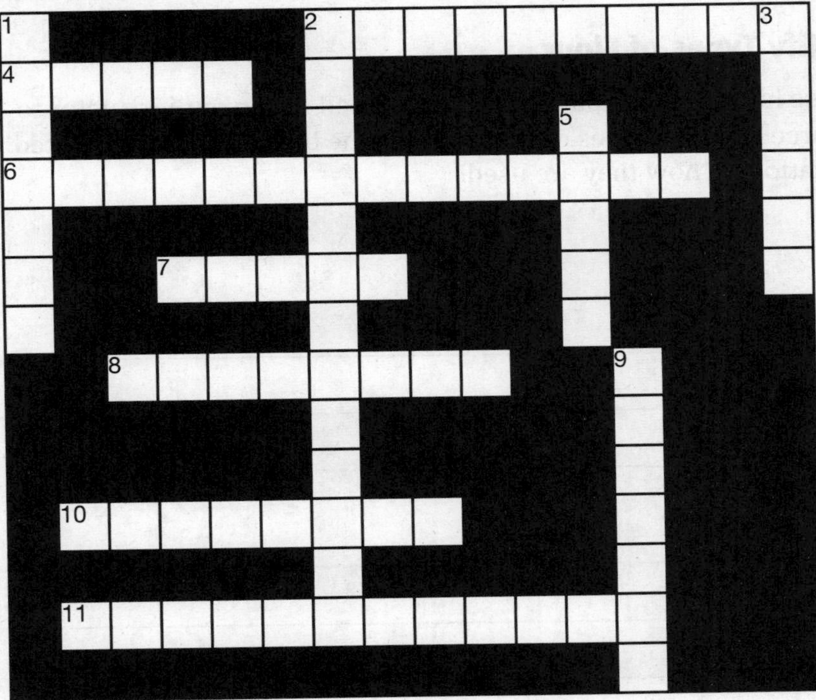

Across

4. Internal texture of a baked product
6. Substance that causes a baked good to rise
7. Contains less liquid than a batter
8. To encircle
10. Shallow, rectangular pan
11. When yeast breaks down sugars into gas

Down

1. Weighing
2. Pan with a releasable bottom
3. Firm, elastic substance that affects texture
5. A living organism necessary for the rising process
9. The process by which moisture is lost

Name ______________________ Date ______________ Class ____________

Chapter 26 Baking Techniques

PROJECT Culinary Review
Bake Quick Breads

Scenario Using the proper ingredients in the bakeshop is vital for baked products to turn out properly. The incorrect ingredients can cause differences in texture and flavor. In this project, you will bake three different quick breads using three different types of flour, and evaluate them for flavor, texture, and appearance.

Academic Skills You Will Use	Culinary Skills You Will Use
SCIENCE **NSES B** Develop an understanding of the structure and properties of matter. **NSES A** Develop abilities necessary to do scientific inquiry.	• Sanitation and safety knowledge • Ingredient knowledge • Baking ingredients and techniques

Step 1 Identify Types of Flour

Directions Use information from your textbook and from your instructor to describe the three different types of flour used in the bakeshop that are listed. Include information on how they are used.

Bread Flour: ______________________________

____

____

____

Cake Flour: ______________________________

____

____

____

Pastry Flour: ______________________________

____

____

____

Name ______________________ Date ______________ Class __________

Chapter 26 Baking Techniques

PROJECT Culinary Review (continued)
Bake Quick Breads

Step 2 Mix Quick Bread Batter

Directions Follow your teacher's instructions to form groups. Use a simple quick bread recipe from your teacher and mix three different quick bread batters: one using bread flour, one using cake flour, and one using pastry flour. Describe the texture and appearance of each batter in the chart.

Quick Bread Batters	
Batter Type	**Texture and Appearance**
Bread Flour	
Cake Flour	
Pastry Flour	

Predict how you think using different flours might affect the final product.

Name ______________________ Date ____________ Class ____________

Chapter 26

Chapter 26 Baking Techniques

PROJECT Culinary Review (continued)
Bake Quick Breads

Step 3 Bake and Evaluate Quick Breads

Directions Once you have made your prediction, bake the three quick breads as a group. When the quick breads are done, evaluate them for flavor, texture, and overall appearance. Write your comments in the chart.

Baked Quick Bread			
Quick Bread Type	**Flavor**	**Texture**	**Overall Appearance**
Bread Flour			
Cake Flour			
Pastry Flour			

What can you learn from this experiment?

____

____

____

____

____

____

____

____

____

____

For additional culinary projects and study tools, visit this book's Online Learning Center at glencoe.com.

Name ________________ Date ________ Class ________

Chapter 27 Yeast Breads and Rolls

Section 27.1 Yeast Dough Basics

NCTE 3 Apply strategies to interpret texts.

English Language Arts Project

Describe Yeast Doughs

Directions Review the information on hard lean doughs, soft medium doughs, sweet rich doughs, and rolled-in fat doughs in Section 27.1 of your textbook. Build your reading comprehension skills by describing the characteristics of each dough in your own words.

Hard Lean Dough

____

____

____

____

____

Soft Medium Dough

____

____

____

____

Sweet Rich Dough

____

____

____

____

____

Rolled-In Fat Dough

____

____

____

____

Chapter 27

Name ______________________ Date ____________ Class ____________

Chapter 27 Yeast Breads and Rolls

Section 27.2 Yeast Dough Production

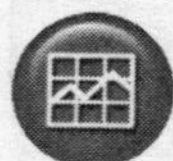

Mathematics Project

Understand Units

NCTM Measurement
Understand measurable attributes of objects and the units, systems, and processes of measurement.

Directions Circle the best answer for each question.

1. Which unit would not be appropriate for measuring the length of a baguette?
   a) meters b) kilometers c) centimeters d) inches

2. Which unit could you use to measure the surface area of a slice of bread?
   a) cubic inches b) cubic feet c) square inches d) centimeters

3. Which unit would be best for measuring the diameter of a spherical dinner roll?
   a) inches b) degrees c) cubic inches d) yards

4. A measurement in cups cannot be converted into:
   a) tablespoons b) grams c) milliliters d) fluid ounces

5. Which unit would you not expect to see in a yeast bread formula?
   a) grams b) pounds c) ounces d) milligrams

6. Which unit would be most appropriate for measuring the volume of a loaf of bread?
   a) square inches b) cubic inches c) cubic meters d) square feet

7. A measurement in kilograms can be converted into
   a) ounces b) cups c) kilometers d) fluid ounces

8. A formula calls for 1 gallon of water. Which of the following is not an acceptable equivalent?
   a) 2 quarts b) 16 cups c) 128 fluid ounces d) 8 pints

Name ______________________ Date ____________ Class ________

Chapter 27 Yeast Breads and Rolls

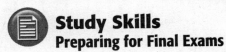

Study Skills
Preparing for Final Exams

Directions Finals week can be a stressful time of year. You can reduce your stress level and still score well on your tests. Read the tips. Then, answer the questions.

Tips to Prepare for Final Exams
• Start studying ahead of time. Do not try to cram an entire semester of material into a day or two before the test. • Each week, review the material you covered in class. Note the material that you feel is important and may be on the final exam. • Keep all of your prior tests and quizzes and use them to review for the final exam. An instructor often will use some of the same test material on the final exam. • During finals week, get plenty of rest. You want to be able to concentrate while studying and while taking the final. • Organize group study sessions with your classmates. This may help alert you to material that you may have overlooked on your own. • Do not put too much pressure on yourself to perform well. Remain as relaxed as possible. Remind yourself that you have prepared properly and will do well on all of your final exams.

1. Why is it important to begin studying finals ahead of time?

____

____

2. Why is it helpful to keep and review prior tests and quizzes when you study for a final?

____

____

____

____

3. List steps that you could take to keep your class materials organized so that you have them available when you begin to study for finals.

____

____

____

____

Name ______________________ Date ______________ Class ________

Chapter 27 Yeast Breads and Rolls

Certification Test Practice
Using Old Tests

Directions Read the tips for using old tests. Then, complete the fill-in-the-blank test. Use the correct terms to fill in the blanks and complete the essay. Not all of the terms will be used.

Chapter 27

Ways to Use Old Tests
You can use old tests to help you prepare for end-of-chapter or end-of-term exams that are cumulative. To use old tests: • Review tests you have already taken that contain material that will appear on an end-of-chapter or end-of-term exam. • Read any teacher's comments on the old tests. • Re-read all the questions and correct answers on the old test. • Correct any questions that you missed. Revise incorrect answers.

starters	hard lean dough	leavens
tempted	sweet rich dough	pan
rolled-in fat yeast dough	proofing	let down
rise	peel	crust
bench rest	shape	rounded
wash	gluten	kneading

Karla was excited about her first day working in a bakeshop. Her day began with a short review of how yeast breads are made. She reviewed how ______________ development is key to the correct texture of a yeast product. In yeast bread, yeast ______________ the bread, causing it to rise. Karla also reviewed information on ______________, which can give breads such as sourdough a unique texture and flavor. When her workday began, Karla was asked to make a ______________ so that the resulting bread would have a relatively dry, chewy crumb and a hard outer ______________. After ______________ the dough and setting it aside to ______________, she began work on a ______________ that would make a yeast-raised coffee cake. Although Karla was ______________ to add a little more flour to make the dough easier to work with, she resisted. Once her first dough had risen, Karla needed to ______________ it into the right form, and ______________ it in the correct loaf pan. She allowed extra time for ______________ the bread, allowing it to rise to its final height before baking. She slashed the top of the loaf with a knife, and placed the bread in the oven. Once the bread was done, she tapped it to test for doneness. She smiled as she looked at the bread—her accomplishments for the day!

Name ______________________ Date ______________ Class __________

Chapter 27 Yeast Breads and Rolls

Content and Academic Vocabulary
English Language Arts

NCTE 12 Use language to accomplish individual purposes.

Directions Write the letter of each vocabulary term on the line next to the definition.

Content Vocabulary		Academic Vocabulary
a. hard lean dough	g. punching	m. tempted
b. soft medium dough	h. shaping	n. notable
c. sweet rich dough	i. panning	o. critical
d. rolled-in fat yeast dough	j. proofing	p. correspond
e. straight-dough method	k. slashing	
f. let down	l. oven spring	

1. ______ Mixing all the ingredients together in a single step
2. ______ The final leavening effort, occurring before internal temperatures become hot enough to kill the yeast cells
3. ______ Well known
4. ______ Combining the fat into the dough through a rolling and folding action
5. ______ A condition in which the ingredients in a dough completely break down
6. ______ Making shallow cuts in the surface of an item, done just before baking
7. ______ To be enticed
8. ______ A dough that incorporates up to 25% of both fat and sugar
9. ______ To match
10. ______ The action of turning the sides of the dough into the middle and turning the dough over
11. ______ Placing in the correct type of pan
12. ______ Necessary
13. ______ Allowing the leavening action of yeast to achieve its final strength before yeast cells are killed by hot oven temperatures
14. ______ Forming the dough into distinctive shapes
15. ______ A dough that produces items with a soft crumb and crust
16. ______ A dough made from flour, water, salt, and yeast that yields products with a relatively dry, chewy crumb

Name ______________________ Date ____________ Class ________

Chapter 27 Yeast Breads and Rolls

PROJECT

Culinary Review
Form and Evaluate Soft Rolls

Scenario Yeast rolls are a part of most restaurant dinners. They can be formed into many appealing shapes. In this project, you will form several different shapes of yeast rolls, bake them, and assess their shape, crust, texture, aroma, and flavor.

Academic Skills You Will Use	Culinary Skills You Will Use
ENGLISH LANGUAGE ARTS **NCTE 5** Use different writing process elements to communicate effectively. **MATHEMATICS** **NCTM Measurement** Apply appropriate techniques, tools, and formulas to determine measurements.	• Sanitation and safety knowledge • Baking skills • Food evaluation

Chapter 27

Step 1 Shape Cloverleaf Rolls

Directions Follow your teacher's instructions to make yeast roll dough, or use dough provided by your teacher. Once the dough is made and has risen, use a dough scraper or bench knife to divide the dough into three equal parts. Then, use the first part to shape cloverleaf rolls using the directions shown.

Cloverleaf Rolls
1. Divide the scaled dough into smaller parts. **2.** Divide the smaller pieces of dough into three equal parts. **3.** Shape the three equal parts into balls. **4.** Place three balls in each cup of a greased muffin tin.

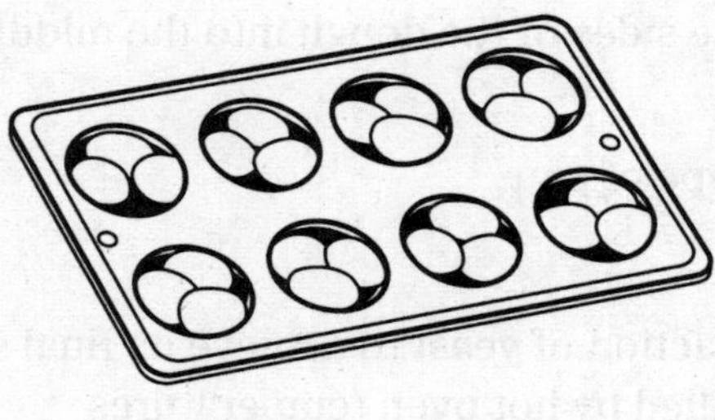

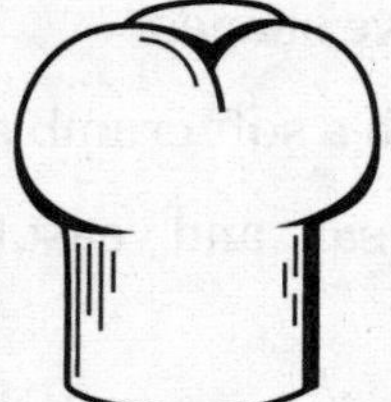

Name ______________________ Date ____________ Class ____________

Chapter 27 Yeast Breads and Rolls

PROJECT Culinary Review (continued)
Form and Evaluate Soft Rolls

Step 2 Shape Parkerhouse and Single-Knotted Rolls

Directions Follow the directions to shape Parkerhouse and single-knotted rolls using the rest of the dough.

Parkerhouse Rolls
1. Divide the scaled dough into three equal portions. 2. Round the dough as shown. 3. Place the ball of dough on a pre-floured bench. 4. Using a rolling pin, flatten only the center of the dough. 5. Fold the flattened dough in half. 6. Using the palm of your hand, press on the folded edge of the dough to make a crease.

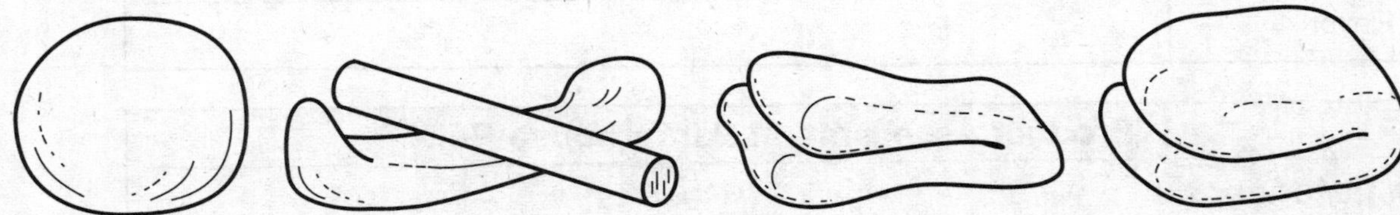

Single-Knotted Rolls
1. Divide the scaled dough into three equal parts. 2. Place the dough on a pre-floured bench. 3. Using the palm of your hand, roll the dough into long, narrow ropes. 4. Cross the bottom end of the rope over the top end of the rope. 5. Tuck the end in the loop.

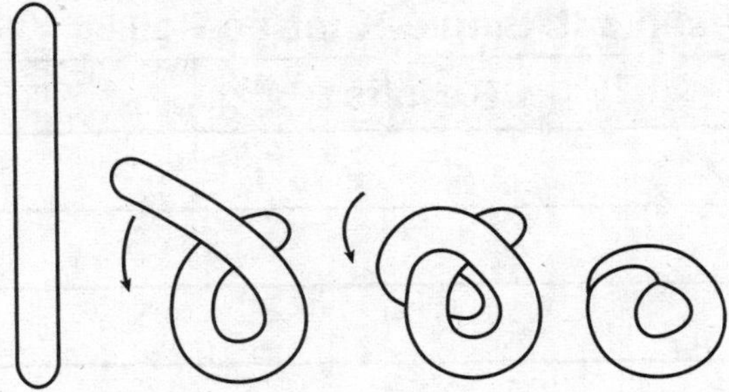

Chapter 27

Chapter 27 Yeast Breads and Rolls

PROJECT Culinary Review (continued)
Form and Evaluate Soft Rolls

Step 3 Bake and Evaluate Rolls

Directions Once you have formed your rolls, bake them and evaluate them, using the charts provided.

Product Assessment: Cloverleaf Rolls	
Category	**Results**
Shape	
Crust	
Texture	
Aroma	
Flavor	

Product Assessment: Parkerhouse Rolls	
Category	**Results**
Shape	
Crust	
Texture	
Aroma	
Flavor	

Product Assessment: Single-Knotted Rolls	
Category	**Results**
Shape	
Crust	
Texture	
Aroma	
Flavor	

For additional culinary projects and study tools, visit this book's Online Learning Center at **glencoe.com**.

Name ______________________ Date __________ Class __________

Chapter 28 Quick Breads

Section 28.1 Making Biscuits

English Language Arts Project

Research Biscuit Recipes

NCTE 8 Use information resources to gather information and create and communicate knowledge.

Directions Use online and print resources to find two recipes that use biscuits as a base. Print a copy of the recipes and attach them to this sheet. Then, answer the questions.

Recipe 1 Name: ______________________

Recipe 2 Name: ______________________

1. What part of a meal is the recipe?

   Recipe 1: ______________________

   Recipe 2: ______________________

2. From what culture does the recipe come?

   Recipe 1: ______________________

   Recipe 2: ______________________

3. How does the recipe use biscuits?

   Recipe 1: ______________________

   Recipe 2: ______________________

4. What flavor and texture does the biscuit give to the recipe?

   Recipe 1: ______________________

   Recipe 2: ______________________

Chapter 28

Name ______________________ Date ______________ Class __________

Chapter 28 Quick Breads

Section 28.2 Making Muffins

Mathematics Project
Cost Muffins

NCTM Number and Operations Compute fluently and make reasonable estimates.

Directions Use the form to calculate the Total Cost, the Cost per Serving, and the Selling Price. Use the formula **Amount + Unit Cost = Extended Cost**. Add the ingredient Extended Costs to find the Total Cost. Then, use the given formulas to calculate the Mark-Up, Selling Price, and Cost per Serving.

Recipe Yield: 15

Cost per Serving: ________

Muffins				
Ingredients	**Amounts**	**Unit Cost**	**Extended Cost**	**Mark-Up = 25%**
Eggs	2	$0.06/each		**Calculate Mark-Up** (Total Cost × Mark Up)
Milk	1 c.	$0.17/c.		
Salad Oil	½ c.	$0.23/c.		**Calculate the Total Selling Price** (Total Cost + Mark-Up)
Flour	3 c.	$0.04/c.		
Sugar	1 c.	$0.23/c.		**Calculate Cost per Serving** (Total Cost ÷ Recipe Yield)
Baking Powder	1 Tbsp., 1 tsp.	$0.03/tsp.		
Salt	1 tsp.	$0.03/tsp.		

Total Cost: ________

Chapter 28

Name ______________________ Date ____________ Class __________

Chapter 28 Quick Breads

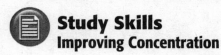

Study Skills
Improving Concentration

Directions Read the tips for improving concentration. Then, follow the prompt to complete a timed exercise about Chapter 28.

How to Improve Your Concentration
Improving your concentration allows you to take in more information at a faster rate. To concentrate better while studying: • Go to your study place. Remove distractions such as the phone and television. • Plan to study for 20 minutes, and then take a break. Repeat this throughout your study period. • Before you begin, take a couple of deep breaths. Say these words in your head as you breathe in: "I breathe in and let go of my thoughts." As you breathe out, say: "I breathe out and relax." • As you study, remind yourself to think about what you are reading. You may be able to concentrate for only a few moments before other thoughts enter your mind. Do not give up. Concentration takes practice. Before you know it, you will be able to concentrate for longer and longer periods of time.

Timed activities demand your concentration. If your mind drifts, you use up valuable time. Practice your concentration skills by taking no more than three minutes to fill in the blanks using the terms in the box.

dry ingredients	biscuit method	leavening agent
fluffy	tenderizer	cornmeal
creaming method	blending method	

Quick breads are breads that do not use yeast as a ________________. They can be plain, lightly glazed, sprinkled with confectioner's sugar, or frosted. Common quick breads are muffins, loaf breads, biscuits, pancakes, scones, and waffles.

There are three methods of making quick breads. The first method, the ________________, involves cutting in fat into flour until the mixture resembles ________________. Then, liquids are added. This method produces a flaky product.

In the ________________, liquid, liquid fat, sugar, and eggs are combined. Then, ________________ are added. The liquid fat and sugar act as a ________________. This makes quick breads such as fruit breads and muffins.

The third method, the ________________, uses solid shortening instead of liquid fat. Bakers use a mixer to cream together softened shortening and sugar. Once the mixture is ________________, eggs are added, one at a time, until mixed in. Then, dry and liquid ingredients are added alternately. Muffins made using this method have a cake-like texture.

Chapter 28

Name ______________________ Date ______________ Class ______________

Chapter 28 Quick Breads

Certification Test Practice

Using Test-Taking Strategies

Directions Read the strategies to use while taking a test. Then, take the test. Complete the questions using short answers.

Test-Taking Strategies
• Read all instructions carefully and make sure you understand them. • Skim the entire test before you start. • Take note of the point values of each section. This will help you pace yourself. • Skip questions you are stuck on and return to them later. You might recall an answer while working on another part of the test. • If you are unsure of the full answer for a question, answer what you know. You might get partial credit.

Chapter 28

1. Why is it important not to overmix biscuits?

____

____

2. Describe the flavor of a good-quality biscuit.

____

____

____

3. How does a muffin get its structure?

____

____

4. What are the characteristics of a well-made loaf bread?

____

____

____

5. What is the proper way to thaw frozen muffin batter?

____

____

____

Name ______________________ Date __________ Class __________

Chapter 28 Quick Breads

Content and Academic Vocabulary
English Language Arts

NCTE 12 Use language to accomplish individual purposes.

Directions Use each vocabulary term to write one sentence that shows you understand the term's meaning. The first one is completed for you.

1. consistency The **consistency** of the pancake batter led Ben to believe he had added too much liquid.
2. deflate ______________________
3. streusel ______________________
4. elastic ______________________
5. deteriorate ______________________
6. biscuit method ______________________
7. potency ______________________
8. aftertaste ______________________
9. separation ______________________
10. pour batter ______________________
11. baking cup ______________________
12. tunnels ______________________
13. drop batter ______________________

Chapter 28

Name ______________________ Date ____________ Class ____________

Chapter 28 Quick Breads

PROJECT Culinary Review
Use Different Blending Methods

Scenario The blending method and the creaming method are two different ways to make quick bread. Results in the final products from the two methods can be different. In this project, you will review the two blending methods, create quick breads using both methods, and evaluate the results.

Academic Skills You Will Use	Culinary Skills You Will Use
SCIENCE **NSES F** Develop an understanding of personal and community health. **MATHEMATICS** **NCTE Measurement** Apply appropriate techniques, tools, and formulas to determine measurements.	• Sanitation and safety knowledge • Mixing methods • Bakeshop techniques

Chapter 28

Step 1 Review Mixing Methods

Directions In the space provided, describe the differences between the blending method and the creaming method for making quick breads.

Blending Method

____

____

____

____

____

____

Creaming Method

____

____

____

____

____

____

Name ______________________ Date ____________ Class ________

Chapter 28 Quick Breads

PROJECT Culinary Review (continued)
Use Different Blending Methods

Step 2 Make Quick Breads

Directions Follow your teacher's directions to form groups. Use formulas provided by your teacher to make two different quick bread products—one using the blending method, and one using the creaming method.

Blending Method Recipe: ______________________

Description of Product: ______________________

____

Blending Method Process
1. Gather ingredients 2. Grease deep pan 3. Scale ingredients 4. Combine liquid ingredients 5. Sift dry ingredients 6. Combine liquid and dry ingredients 7. Mix the batter 8. Scale the batter 9. Bake the batter 10. Cool the loaf bread

Creaming Method Recipe: ______________________

Description of Product: ______________________

____

Creaming Method Process
1. Gather ingredients 2. Grease the pan 3. Scale ingredients 4. Sift the dry ingredients 5. Combine solid fat and sugar 6. Add eggs, one at a time 7. Alternately add dry and liquid ingredients 8. Portion batter 9. Bake batter 10. Cool baked product

Chapter 28

Name ______________________ Date ______________ Class ______________

Chapter 28 Quick Breads

PROJECT Culinary Review (continued)
Use Different Blending Methods

Step 3 Assess Quality

Directions Once your quick bread products are baked, evaluate them as a group using the charts.

Blending Method Product Assessment	
Category	**Results**
Shape	
Crust	
Texture	
Aroma	
Flavor	

Creaming Method Product Assessment	
Category	**Results**
Shape	
Crust	
Texture	
Aroma	
Flavor	

For additional culinary projects and study tools, visit this book's Online Learning Center at glencoe.com.

Name ____________________ Date __________ Class __________

Chapter 29 Desserts

Section 29.1 Cookies

Culinary Skills Project
Summarize a Cookie Recipe

Directions Choose a cookie recipe and attach a copy of the recipe to this page. Use the space provided to evaluate the ingredients, equipment, and timing that will be needed to prepare this recipe.

Recipe Name: ____________________

Ingredients: ____________________

Mixing Method: ____________________

Equipment: ____________________

Timing: ____________________

Chapter 29

Name ______________________ Date ______________ Class ______________

Chapter 29 Desserts

Section 29.2 Cakes

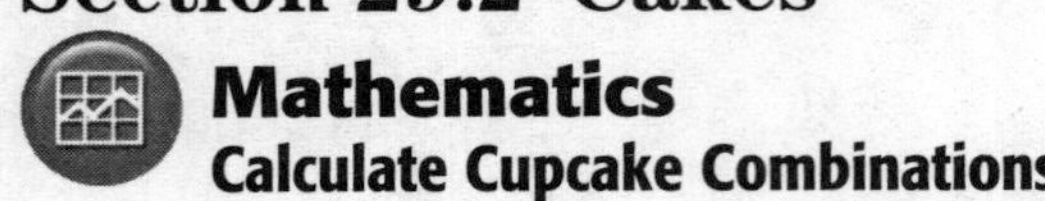

Mathematics
Calculate Cupcake Combinations

NCTM Number and Operations Understand meanings of operations and how they relate to one another.

Directions A permutation is an ordered arrangement of a group of items. A combination is like a permutation, except that the order of the items does not matter. Use the following formulas to answer the questions below. The formulas assume that you are choosing *r* items out of *n* total items. Remember that the "!" stands for "factorial," which is the product of all sequential integers between 1 and *n*. For example, $4! = 4 \times 3 \times 2 \times 1$.

	Permutations	Combinations
Items can be picked more than once	n^r	$\frac{(n + r - 1)!}{r!(n - 1)!}$
Items can NOT be repeated	$\frac{n!}{(n - r)!}$	$\frac{n!}{r!(n - r)!}$

Assume that Laura's cupcake shop sells five different varieties of cupcakes: chocolate (C), vanilla (V), red velvet (R), banana (B), and peanut butter (P).

1. A customer phones in an order for four cupcakes without specifying the flavors. How many different ways can Laura arrange four cupcakes in a to-go box that has four spaces?

____

2. What is the answer to Question 1 if the customer requested that there were no duplicates?

____

3. Levi walks into Laura's shop and wants to order two cupcakes. How many different options does he have?

____

4. List out each option in Question 3 by initial (e.g., write "CV" for chocolate and vanilla). Does this match your answer above?

____

5. What is the answer to Question 3 if Levi did not want two of the same flavor?

____

Name ______________________ Date ______________ Class ______________

Chapter 29 Desserts

Section 29.3 Pies

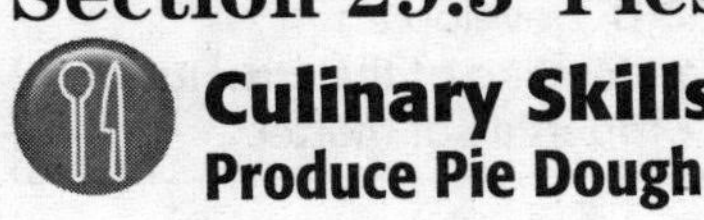

Culinary Skills
Produce Pie Dough

Directions Working in terms, prepare basic pie dough by following the recipe on page 768 of your textbook. Use the pie dough to prepare the pie of your choice. After making your pie, answer the questions in complete sentences.

1. Explain the purpose of salt in pie dough.

____

____

____

2. Predict what will happen if your pie crust is overmixed. Explain your prediction.

____

____

____

3. Explain why dusting your pie crust with the right amount of flour is important to the quality of the pie crust.

____

____

____

____

4. Explain why pastry flour is used for pie crusts, instead of bread flour.

____

____

____

5. How can you safely freeze pie dough for later use?

____

____

____

____

Chapter 29

Name ______________________ Date ______________ Class ______________

Chapter 29 Desserts

Section 29.4 Specialty Desserts

Science Project

Research Gelatin

NSES B Develop an understanding of the structure and properties of matter.

Directions Use the Internet and other print resources to research gelatin, and then answer the questions below.

1. Explain how gelatin is formed and where it comes from.

____

____

____

____

2. Explain the process of gelatinization of starches.

____

____

____

____

3. Explain the common uses of gelatin in food.

____

____

____

____

4. Explain how gelatin is different from agar-agar and pectin.

____

____

____

____

____

____

____

Chapter 29

Name ______________________ Date ____________ Class ________

Chapter 29 Desserts

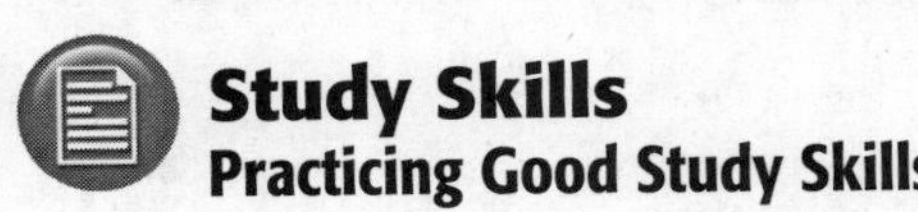

Study Skills
Practicing Good Study Skills

Directions Read the tips for practicing good study habits. Then, follow the prompt.

How to Practice Good Study Habits
• Review class material every day instead of cramming it all in just before a test. • Be alert in class and take good notes. • Complete all assignments given by your teacher. • Study with classmates to make learning more fun and active. • Maintain an organization notebook and folder for each separate subject. • Ask your instructor if you do not understand certain material. • Keep the television or radio off while studying. • Get plenty of sleep each night so you can better concentrate on your studies.

Organization is one facet of good study habits. Studying is easier when school subjects are arranged in separate notebooks and folders. After reading Chapter 29, use critical thinking skills to give three specific examples of how you think organization can help people plan desserts better.

1. Plan a batch of cookies ______________________________

2. Plan a cake ______________________________

3. Substitute an ingredient in a pie for one that you do not have in stock.

Chapter 29

Name ______________________ Date ______________ Class __________

Chapter 29 Desserts

Certification Test Practice

Rewarding Yourself

Directions Read the tips for rewarding yourself. Then, take the sample true/false test. When the answer is a false statement, write the truth.

How to Reward Yourself
If you reward yourself for studying and meeting academic goals, you will find the process more enjoyable, To reward yourself, do the following: • When studying for a test, take a 10-minute break every hour. Reward yourself with a short call to a friend, playtime with a pet, or a healthy treat. • Throughout your study session, take mini-breaks lasting one minute. During these breaks, close your eyes, stretch, and take a few deep breaths. • Set goals for how much time you would like to spend studying on a given day. If you meet your goal, reward yourself at the end of your study session. • Set a goal for how well you would like to do on a test. If you take a test and meet your goal, reward yourself with a fun activity with friends.

1. The crispiness of a cookie is influenced by the type of fat, flour, and sugar, and the amount of liquid and baking soda that are used when baking them. T F

____

____

2. Chiffon cakes have less saturated fat and cholesterol than any cake but angel food cake. T F

____

____

3. Unlike creaming method cakes, blending method cakes can be scaled by weight or volume. T F

____

____

4. Water or milk at 90°F (32°C) will allow pie dough to form gluten as it is mixed with flour. T F

____

____

5. Panning is a manner of decorating a pie crust by making uniform folds around the edge of the pie at the pan's brim. T F

____

____

Chapter 29

Name ______________________ Date ______________ Class ________

Chapter 29 Desserts

Content and Academic Vocabulary
English Language Arts

NCTE 12 Use language to accomplish individual purposes.

Directions Write the correct content or academic vocabulary term in the line next to the definition. You will not use all of the terms.

Content Vocabulary		Academic Vocabulary
spread	flaky dough	turn
one-stage method	mealy dough	deal
pound cake	baking blind	contrast
sponge cake	sherbet	substituted
meringue	custard	
fondant	sundae	

_______________ As a comparison

_______________ A dessert that contains a pound each of butter, flour, sugar, and eggs

_______________ A mixture of sugar, water, and flavorings that serves as a base for icings

_______________ Pie dough that resembles coarse cornmeal

_______________ A frozen dessert that combines fruit juices, sugar, water, and a little cream or milk

_______________ A dessert that contains one or more scoops of ice cream topped with garnishes, fruits, or syrups

_______________ Switched; replaced

_______________ An airy, light-textured cake

_______________ Whipped egg whites

_______________ Baking pie shells in advance

_______________ A dessert made of eggs, milk or cream, flavorings, and sweeteners, either baked or cooked in a double boiler

_______________ To become; to change or transform

_______________ A process in which all ingredients are mixed in a single stage

Name ______________________ Date ____________ Class ________

Chapter 29 Desserts

PROJECT Culinary Review
Bake Pies

Scenario Any kind of baking project should be planned ahead of time to produce proper results. In this project, you will work in teams to research, plan and prepare pies to submit for a class competition.

Academic Skills You Will Use	Culinary Skills You Will Use
SCIENCE **NSES F** Develop an understanding of personal and community health. **MATHEMATICS** **NCTE Measurement** Apply appropriate techniques, tools, and formulas to determine measurements.	• Sanitation and safety knowledge • Thermometer use • Baking skills

Step 1 Research a Pie

Directions Following your teacher's instructions, form four teams with your classmates. Each team will prepare an apple, cherry, chocolate, or coconut cream pie. Each team should prepare a different type of pie.

1. Use the Internet or print resources to research your pie. Describe the ingredients, the baking process, and how the final product should taste and look.

____

____

____

____

____

____

____

____

____

____

____

____

____

____

Chapter 29

Name ______________________ Date ______________ Class ______________

Chapter 29 Desserts

PROJECT Culinary Review (continued)
Bake Pies

Step 2 Form a Work Plan

Directions Create a work plan for your project. Divide the tasks equally among team members. Write the steps, actions, and estimated times in the chart.

Team Member Names

____

Team Leader

____

Step	Action to Be Taken	Estimated Time to Complete	Actual Time to Complete
1			
2			
3			
4			
5			
6			
7			
8			

Name ______________________ Date ____________ Class ________

Chapter 29 Desserts

PROJECT Culinary Review (continued)
Bake Pies

Step 3 Bake Your Pie and Evaluate Your Process

Directions Follow the work plan you created in Step 2 to bake your pie. Record the actual amount of time needed for each step in the chart. Then, evaluate how effective your work plan was.

1. Prepare your team's pie as directed in the formula. Use the following mathematical formula to convert the yield of the recipe if needed.

   Step 1 desired yield ÷ existing yield = conversion factor

   Step 2 existing quantity × conversion factor = desired quantity

   ____

   ____

2. Are there any parts of the process on which you can improve? Did you accurately estimate the time it would take to prepare and bake your pie? How can you improve the process?

   ____

   ____

   ____

   ____

   ____

   ____

   ____

   ____

   ____

   ____

   ____

   ____

   ____

For additional culinary projects and study tools, visit this book's Online Learning Center at glencoe.com.

Chapter 29

Name ______________________ Date ______________ Class __________

COMPETITIVE EVENTS PRACTICE

Bake an Angel Food Cake

Directions Follow your teacher's instructions to form competition teams of two to four people. Each team will be given a formula for an angel food cake, and will make an angel food cake using that formula. Special attention should be paid to the quality of the baked product.

Judging
In this competition, you will be judged on:
• How well your team follows the formula • The appearance and flavor of your angel food cake • The sanitation procedures you follow • The cleanliness of your workspace

Preparation Phase

1. Write a list of the characteristics of a good-quality angel food cake. Turn in a copy of your list to your teacher.

 ____

 ____

 ____

2. Prepare your workspace for competition. During preparation:
   - Retrieve all necessary equipment and tools
   - Observe all safety and sanitation procedures
   - Scale all ingredients
   - Use a sanitizing solution to clean your workspace before beginning

   Do not prepare any part of the cake at this time.

Cooking Phase

1. Make your angel food cake, using the list you created as a guide for results. Make sure to plate your cake creatively. Do not cut the cake once it is finished. It should be sent to the judge whole. You will have 1½ hours to make your cake.

2. Bring your cake to the tasting area designated by your teacher when it is completed and ready for judging, or at the end of the time period. Display your cake with the cake description you wrote earlier.

COMPETITIVE EVENTS PRACTICE (continued)

Competitive Events Review

Once the competition has been completed, write a short essay on the experience of competing with other teams. How important is mixing to the success of a cake? What did you do in your preparation steps to ensure a good final product? What would you have done differently next time?

Food Safety Rules

Food safety is everyone's responsibility. Remember these general food safety rules. You can learn to keep food fresh and safe and to keep everyone healthy.

Wash Hands Properly Wash your hands with hot running water and soap for at least 15 seconds. Scrub the front and back of your hands, between your fingers, and under your fingernails. Rinse off soap with hot running water. Dry your hands well with a clean towel or air dryer. Use a paper towel to turn off the water faucet.

Avoid Spreading Bacteria Do not handle other people's food if you are sick. Cover an open cut or sore on your hands with a clean waterproof bandage. Cover your nose and mouth with clean tissue when you sneeze or cough. Handle food with clean utensils. Tie back any long hair before preparing food. Wear clean clothes and roll up the sleeves. Wear a clean apron. Use a clean spoon for each tasting. Do not taste foods containing raw or partly cooked meat, poultry, fish, or eggs.

Keep the Kitchen Clean Use a disinfectant, a mixture of chlorine bleach and water, or hot, soapy water to clean kitchen surfaces. Wipe up spills right away. Sweep the floor whenever needed. Keep dirty dishes, pots, and pans away from food preparation areas. Wash dirty dishes immediately in hot soapy water and rinse in hot water. Clean the can opener after each use. Use different towels for drying dishes and your hands. Keep kitchen garbage in a tightly covered can.

Avoid Cross-Contamination Keep raw meat, poultry, fish, and their juices away from ready-to-eat foods. If possible, keep one cutting board just for raw meat, poultry, and fish. Wash everything that touches raw food before reusing it. Use paper towels to wipe up food scraps, spills, or meat juices. Then, wash the counter and your hands right away.

Thaw and Cook Food Properly Never thaw food at room temperature. Cook food fully. Check internal temperature with a clean meat thermometer. Avoid raw or partly cooked eggs. Keep foods out of the temperature danger zone (41°F to 135°F; 5°C to 57°C).

Safety in the Kitchen

Accidents in the kitchen can happen—but they are easily prevented. The main cause of kitchen accidents is carelessness. Remember the following rules to help prevent accidents:

Basic Kitchen Safety Rules

For General Safety Pay attention to the task. Use the right tool for the job. Do not let hair, jewelry, or clothing dangle. They could catch fire or get tangled in equipment.

To Prevent Cuts Store knives in a container or block designed for them. Do not soak any sharp utensils in a sink where you may not see them. Always use a cutting board. Clean up broken glass carefully using a broom and dustpan for big pieces, and a wet paper towel for glass dust.

To Prevent Falls and Other Injuries Keep drawers and doors closed. Wipe up spills, splatters, and peelings on the floor immediately. Use a sturdy stool to reach higher shelves. Store heavy items within easy reach.

To Prevent Electrical Shock Keep small electrical appliances away from water. Keep cords away from heat sources. Unplug small appliances before cleaning them and do not immerse them in water. Do not plug too many appliances into one outlet. Keep utensils such as forks out of toasters and other electrical appliances.

To Prevent Burns Keep potholders within easy reach and use them to handle hot items. Turn the handles of pots and pans toward the inside of the range to prevent accidental spills. Carefully lift the cover of a hot pan to prevent steam from burning you. Wait until a spill cools before wiping it up.

To Prevent Fires Keep flammable items away from the range. Watch foods as they cook on the range. Store aerosol cans away from heat. Keep a fire extinguisher at hand and know how to use it.

To Prevent Accidental Poisoning Store all household chemicals away from food and out of children's reach. Keep chemicals in a locked cabinet if possible and clearly labeled. Follow label directions when you use household chemicals.

Tr = Trace amount
*1 RE = 3.33 IU from animal foods or 1 mcg retinol
1 RE = 10 IU from plant foods or 6 mcg beta carotene.

Item No.	Food Description	Approximate Measure	Weight	Food energy	Protein	Fat	Cholesterol	Calcium	Iron	Sodium	Vitamin A value*	Vitamin C
				Nutrients in Indicated Quantity								
			Grams	Calories	Grams	Grams	Milligrams	Milligrams	Milligrams	Milligrams	Retinol equivalents	Milligrams
	Beverages											
9	Club soda	12 fl oz	355	0	0	0	0	18	Tr	75	0	0
10	Regular cola	12 fl oz	369	137	Tr	Tr	0	7	0.4	15	0	0
11	Diet, artificially sweetened cola	12 fl oz	355	7	Tr	Tr	0	11	0.4	28	0	0
20	Fruit punch drink	8 fl oz	248	119	0	0	0	20	0.2	25	0	1
	Dairy Product											
	Natural Cheese											
32	Cheddar, cut pieces	1 oz	28	114	7	9	30	205	0.2	176	75	0
38	Cottage cheese, lowfat (2%)	1 cup	226	163	28	2	9	138	0.3	918	25	0
43	Mozzarella, part skim milk	1 oz	28	86	7	6	15	208	Tr	150	39	0
46	Parmesan, grated	1 tbsp	5	22	2	1	4	55	Tr	76	6	0
52	Pasteurized process American cheese	1 oz	28	105	6	9	26	155	Tr	417	71	0
	Milk, fluid:											
78	Whole (3.3% fat)	1 cup	244	146	8	8	24	276	Tr	98	68	0
79	Reduced fat (2%)	1 cup	244	122	8	5	20	285	Tr	100	134	1
83	Nonfat (skim)	1 cup	247	86	8	Tr	5	504	0.1	128	338	3
85	Buttermilk	1 cup	245	98	8	2	10	284	0.1	257	17	2
88	Evaporated skim milk	1 cup	245	100	10	Tr	5	372	0.4	149	149	2
91	Dried, nonfat, instantized	1 cup	245	81	8	Tr	5	284	Tr	130	162	1
	Milk beverages:											
94	Chocolate milk, low-fat (1%)	1 cup	250	158	8	3	8	288	0.6	152	145	2
105	Shakes, thick; Vanilla	10 oz	283	379	8	13	48	275	0.3	133	133	8
	Milk desserts, frozen:											
	Ice cream, vanilla, regular (about 11% fat):											
107	Hardened	1 cup	133	267	5	14	53	168	0.2	98	146	1
109	Frozen yogurt	1 cup	200	214	9	3	10	318	0.5	120	24	1
	Ice cream, vanilla, low-fat:											
113	Hardened (about 4% fat)	1 cup	131	216	6	6	35	211	0.3	97	168	2
116	Sherbet (about 2% fat)	1 cup	193	278	2	4	0	104	0.3	89	19	11
	Yogurt, made with low-fat milk:											
117	Fruit-flavored	8 oz	245	250	11	3	10	372	0.2	142	24	2
118	Plain	8 oz	245	154	13	4	15	448	0.2	172	34	2

Nutritive Value of Foods Appendix

Nutritive Value of Foods Appendix

Source: USDA Home and Garden Bulletin No. 72, "Nutritive Value of Foods"

Eggs												
	Eggs, large (24 oz. per dozen):											
124	Fried in margarine	1 egg	46	89	6	7	210	26	0.9	238	88	0
125	Hard-cooked, shell removed	1 egg	50	77	6	5	211	25	0.6	139	84	0
Fats and Oils												
129	Butter (4 sticks per lb) (⅛ stick)	1 tbsp	14	102	Tr	12	31	3	0.0	82	97	0
138	Margarine (⅛ stick)	1 tbsp	14	100	Tr	11	0	0	Tr	93	116	0
147	Corn oil	1 cup	218	1,927	0	218	0	0	0.0	0	0	0
	Salad dressings, commercial:											
162	French, Regular	1 tbsp	16	60	Tr	6	1	3	Tr	197	2	0
163	French, Low calorie	1 tbsp	16	24	Tr	2	1	3	0.1	179	2	0
Fish and Shellfish												
177	Fish sticks, frozen, reheated (stock, 4 by 1 by ½ in.)	1 fish stick	28	70	3	4	9	7	0.3	118	9	0
181	Haddock, breaded, fried	3 oz	85	151	16	7	57	44	1.2	105	14	0
182	halibut, broiled, with butter and lemon juice	3 oz	85	113	19	4	48	19	0.4	354	34	3
195	Tuna, canned, oil packed, chunk light	3 oz	85	168	25	7	15	11	1.2	301	20	0
196	Tuna, canned, water-pack, solid white	3 oz	85	99	22	1	26	9	1.3	287	14	0
Fruits and Fruit Juices												
198	Apples, raw, unpeeled, 2¾-in. diam.	1 apple	138	72	Tr	Tr	0	8	0.2	1	4	6
202	Apple juice, bottled or canned	1 cup	248	117	Tr	Tr	0	17	0.9	7	0	28
204	Applesauce, canned, unsweetened	1 cup	244	105	Tr	Tr	0	7	0.3	5	2	3
215	Bananas, raw, without peel, whole	1 banana	118	105	1	Tr	0	6	0.3	1	4	10
229	Fruit cocktail, canned, juice pack	1 cup	237	109	1	Tr	0	19	0.5	9	36	6
230	Grapefruit, raw, without peel, 3¾-in. diam.	½ grapefruit	128	41	1	Tr	0	15	0.1	0	59	44
233	Grapefruit juice, canned, unsweetened	1 cup	247	94	1	Tr	0	17	0.5	2	0	72
237	Grapes, Thompson Seedless	10 grapes	50	30	Tr	Tr	0	0	Tr	0	0	15
239	Grape juice, canned or bottled	1 cup	253	154	1	Tr	0	23	0.6	8	0	Tr
242	Kiwi fruit, raw, without skin	1 kiwifruit	76	46	1	Tr	0	26	0.2	2	3	71
250	Mangos, raw, without skin and seed	1 mango	207	135	1	1	0	21	0.3	4	79	57
251	Cantaloupe	1 melon	814	277	7	2	0	73	1.7	130	1,376	300
253	Nectarines, raw, without pits	1 nectarine	136	60	1	Tr	0	8	0.4	0	23	7
254	Oranges, raw, whole	1 orange	131	62	1	Tr	0	52	0.1	0	14	70
260	Orange juice, frozen concentrate, diluted	1 cup	249	112	2	Tr	0	27	0.3	5	12	98
262	Papayas, raw, ½-in. cubes	1 cup	140	55	1	Tr	0	34	0.1	4	77	87
263	Peaches, raw, whole, 2½-in.diam.	1 peach	98	38	1	Tr	0	6	0.2	0	16	7
273	Pears, raw, with skin, cored, Bartlett, 2½-in. diam.	1 pear	166	96	1	1	0	15	0.3	2	2	7
283	Pineapple, chunks or tidbits, juice pack	1 cup	249	149	1	Tr	0	35	0.7	2	5	24

Tr = Trace amount
*1 RE = 3.33 IU from animal foods or 1 mcg retinol
1 RE = 10 IU from plant foods or 6 mcg beta carotene.

Item No.	Food Description	Approximate Measure	Weight	Food energy	Protein	Fat	Cholesterol	Calcium	Iron	Sodium	Vitamin A value*	Vitamin C
				Nutrients in Indicated Quantity								
			Grams	Calories	Grams	Grams	Milligrams	Milligrams	Milligrams	Milligrams	Retinol equivalents	Milligrams
287	Plantains, without peel, cooked, boiled, sliced	1 cup	190	220	2	Tr	0	4	1.1	10	86	21
288	Plums, raw, 2⅛-in. diam.	1 plum	66	30	Tr	Tr	0	4	0.1	0	11	6
297	Raisins, seedless, cup, not pressed down	1 cup	145	434	5	Tr	0	72	2.7	16	0	3
303	Strawberries, raw, capped, whole	1 cup	144	46	1	Tr	0	23	0.6	1	1	85
309	Watermelon, 4 by 8 in. wedge	1 piece	286	86	2	Tr	0	20	0.7	3	80	23
	Grain Products											
311	Bagels, plain or water, enriched	1 bagel	69	177	7	1	0	61	4.1	309	0	1
314	Biscuits, from mix, 2 in. diameter	1 biscuit	30	97	2	4	2	54	0.6	274	7	Tr
	Breads:											
319	Cracked-wheat bread (18 per loaf)	1 slice	26	68	2	1	0	27	0.9	138	0	0
332	Pita bread, enriched, white, 6½-in. diam.	1 pita	85	234	8	1	0	73	2.2	456	0	0
346	White bread, enriched (18 per loaf)	1 slice	26	69	2	1	0	39	0.9	177	0	0
353	Whole-wheat bread (16 per loaf)	1 slice	29	80	3	1	0	23	1.1	172	0	0
355	Bread stuffing, dry type, from mix	1 cup	140	246	4	12	0	41	1.5	720	109	0
	Breakfast cereals:											
359	Cream of Wheat®, cooked	1 cup	241	106	3	Tr	0	94	8.0	431	0	0
367	Cheerios®	1 oz	30	111	4	2	0	122	10.3	213	150	6
368	Kellogg's® Corn Flakes	1 oz	25	90	2	Tr	0	15	6.7	197	136	5
383	Shredded Wheat	1 oz	25	84	3	1	0	12	0.7	2	0	3
386	Sugar Frosted Flakes, Kellogg's®	1 oz	31	114	1	Tr	0	2	4.5	148	160	6
390	Wheaties®	1 oz	30	106	3	1	0	0	8.1	218	150	6
	Cakes prepared from cake mixes:											
394	Angelfood, 1/12 of cake	1 piece	57	143	3	Tr	0	47	0.1	283	0	0
396	Coffeecake, crumb, 1/12 of 8" cake	1 piece	42	136	3	4	40	47	0.7	181	15	0
398	Devil's food with chocolate frosting, 1/12 of cake	1 piece	109	405	4	16	31	102	2.7	289	61	0
	Cookies, commercial:											
424	Brownies with nuts and frosting	1 brownie	34	129	2	5	12	11	1.1	50	2	0
426	Chocolate chip, 2¼ in. diam.	4 cookies	30	147	2	7	0	10	1.1	89	0	0
429	Fig bars, square, 1⅝-in. square	4 cookies	64	224	2	2	0	40	1.8	224	0	4
430	Oatmeal with raisins, 2⅝-in. diam.	4 cookies	30	135	2	5	0	11	0.7	115	2	Tr
437	Corn chips	1-oz pkg.	28	145	2	8	0	46	0.4	172	0	0
	Crackers:											

Nutritive Value of Foods Appendix

Nutritive Value of Foods Appendix

Source: USDA Home and Garden Bulletin No. 72, "Nutritive Value of Foods"

444	Graham, plain, 2½-in. square	2 crackers	14	59	1	1	0	3	0.5	85	0	0
448	Snack-type, standard	1 cracker	3	15	Tr	1	0	4	0.1	25	0	0
449	Wheat, thin	4 crackers	8	36	1	2	0	4	Tr	64	0	0
	Doughnuts, made with enriched flour:											
456	Cake type, plain, 3¼-in. diam.	1 doughnut	25	105	1	6	9	11	0.5	136	10	0
457	Yeast-leavened, glazed, 3¾-in. diam.	1 doughnut	60	242	4	14	4	26	1.2	205	2	Tr
458	English muffins, plain, enriched	1 muffin	58	132	5	1	0	95	2.3	246	0	1
461	Macaroni, enriched, cooked	1 cup	140	220	8	1	0	10	1.9	325	0	0
	Muffins, 2½-in. diam., commercial mix:											
467	Blueberry	1 muffin	66	183	4	4	20	38	1.1	295	15	1
468	Bran	1 muffin	58	127	5	1	0	54	3.1	183	39	0
470	Noodles (egg noodles), enriched, cooked	1 cup	160	219	7	3	46	19	2.3	378	10	0
	Pancakes, 4-in. diam.:											
474	Plain mix (with enriched flour), egg, milk, oil added	1 pancake	29	65	2	2	5	21	0.6	146	19	Tr
	Pies, 9-in. diam.:											
478	Apple, ⅛ of pie	1 piece	150	356	3	17	0	16	0.7	399	48	5
488	Lemon meringue, ⅛ of pie	1 piece	137	367	2	12	62	77	0.8	200	70	4
494	Pumpkin, ⅛ of pie	1 piece	155	316	2	14	65	146	1.9	349	660	3
	Popcorn, popped:											
497	Air-popped, unsalted	1 cup	8	31	1	Tr	0	1	0.3	1	1	0
498	Popped in vegetable oil, salted	1 cup	11	55	1	3	0	1	0.3	97	0	0
499	Sugar syrup coated	1 cup	35	135	2	1	0	2	0.5	Tr	3	0
500	Pretzels	10 twists	60	229	5	2	0	22	1.0	1,029	0	0
	Rice:											
503	Brown, cooked, served hot	1 cup	195	214	5	2	0	20	0.8	587	0	0
505	White, enriched, cooked, served hot	1 cup	158	204	4	Tr	0	16	1.9	577	0	0
	Rolls, enriched, commercial:											
509	Dinner, 2½-in.diam.	1 roll	28	87	3	2	1	50	1.0	150	0	Tr
510	Frankfurter and hamburger	1 roll	43	120	4	2	0	59	1.4	206	0	0
514	Spaghetti, enriched, cooked	1 cup	140	220	8	1	0	10	1.9	325	0	0
	Legumes, Nuts, and Seeds											
526	Almonds, shelled, whole	1 oz	28	162	6	14	0	69	1.2	0	0	0
	Beans, dry, cooked, drained:											
527	Black	1 cup	177	312	12	15	0	64	2.3	414	0	0
528	Great Northern	1 cup	180	356	16	15	0	149	6.1	356	0	0
531	Pinto	1 cup	178	313	12	15	0	57	2.4	352	0	2
536	Black-eyed peas, dry, cooked (with cooking liquid)	1 cup	224	419	11	20	20	36	3.6	844	0	Tr

Item No.	Food Description	Approximate Measure	Weight	Food energy	Protein	Fat	Cholesterol	Calcium	Iron	Sodium	Vitamin A value*	Vitamin C
			Grams	Calories	Grams	Grams	Milligrams	Milligrams	Milligrams	Milligrams	Retinol equivalents	Milligrams
544	Chickpeas, cooked, drained	1 cup	169	399	15	18	0	74	3.8	409	2	2
550	Lentils, dry, cooked, with peanuts	1 cup	196	323	16	13	0	35	6.1	431	0	3
553	Mixed nuts, dry roasted, salted	1 oz	28	173	5	16	0	30	0.9	111	0	1
555	Peanuts, roasted in oil, salted	1 cup	144	863	40	76	0	88	2.2	461	0	1
557	Peanut butter	1 tbsp	16	94	4	8	0	7	0.3	73	0	0
564	Refried beans, canned	1 cup	253	367	16	13	15	96	4.2	711	0	10
	Soy Products:											
567	Miso	1 cup	275	547	32	17	0	157	6.9	10,252	11	0
568	Tofu, piece 2¼ by 2¾ by 1 in.	1 piece	124	76	8	5	0	138	1.4	10	0	Tr
569	Sunflower seeds, dry, hulled	1 oz	28	162	7	14	0	33	1.9	1	1	Tr
570	Tahini	1 tbsp	15	89	3	8	0	64	1.3	17	0	0
	Meat and Meat Products											
	Beef, cooked:											
	Braised or pot roasted:											
575	Chuck blade. lean and fat, piece	3 oz	85	258	24	17	80	10	2.5	189	0	0
577	Round, bottom, lean and fat piece	3 oz	85	190	29	8	84	7	2.3	37	0	0
578	Lean only from item 577	3 oz	85	144	24	5	61	5	2.0	32	0	0
580	Ground beef, regular, broiled, patty	4 oz	85	235	22	16	75	26	2.0	340	0	0
585	Round, eye of, lean and fat, roasted	3 oz	85	143	25	4	46	6	2.0	32	0	0
587	Sirloin, steak, broiled, lean and fat	3 oz	85	214	23	13	70	14	1.6	317	0	0
590	Beef, dried, chipped	2.5 oz	71	109	22	1	56	4	2.1	1,981	0	0
	Lamb:											
593	Chops, loin, broiled, lean and fat	4 oz	72	226	16	18	68	14	1.4	281	0	0
	Pork, cured, cooked:											
599	Bacon, regular	3 slices	16	87	6	7	18	2	0.2	370	2	0
601	Ham, light cure, roasted, lean and fat	3 oz	85	137	17	7	54	7	0.6	936	9	0
	Luncheon meat:											
605	Chopped ham (8 slices per 6-oz pkg.)	1 slice	28	45	5	2	15	2	0.3	358	0	0
	Pork, fresh, cooked:											
610	Chop, loin, pan fried, lean and fat	3 oz	44	123	12	8	35	10	0.4	169	1	Tr
614	Rib, roasted, lean and fat	3 oz	85	279	20	22	78	21	0.9	44	3	Tr
	Sausages:											

Tr = Trace amount
*1 RE = 3.33 IU from animal foods or 1 mcg retinol
1 RE = 10 IU from plant foods or 6 mcg beta carotene.

Nutritive Value of Foods Appendix

Nutritive Value of Foods Appendix

Source: USDA Home and Garden Bulletin No. 72, "Nutritive Value of Foods"

618	Bologna, slice (8 per 8-oz pkg.)	1 slice	28	86	4	7	17	24	0.3	206	7	Tr
620	Brown and serve, browned	1 link	13	44	2	4	7	2	0.2	150	0	0
621	Frankfurter, cooked (reheated)	1	57	176	8	15	43	28	1.0	712	5	0
Mixed Dishes												
629	Beef and vegetable stew, home recipe	1 cup	249	182	25	5	42	47	2.5	817	271	7
631	Chicken a la king, home recipe	1 cup	241	460	25	33	190	142	1.9	952	323	5
642	Spaghetti in tomato sauce with cheese, home recipe	1 cup	248	293	10	4	0	40	2.7	563	32	4
Fast Foods												
645	Cheeseburger, regular	1 sandwich	107	317	17	15	46	164	2.8	547	29	0
648	English muffin, egg, cheese, bacon	1 sandwich	135	382	21	19	247	258	3.7	932	140	1
649	Fish sandwich, regular, with cheese	1 sandwich	207	596	27	30	72	286	4.2	1,176	43	Tr
651	Hamburger, regular	1 sandwich	93	270	15	11	34	86	2.7	369	0	0
653	Pizza, cheese, 1/8 of 12-in. diam.	1 slice	86	237	11	10	21	181	1.6	462	68	Tr
654	Roast beef sandwich	1 sandwich	136	341	27	14	67	86	4.3	602	0	0
655	Taco	1 taco	76	98	7	3	50	64	0.9	306	9	3
Poultry and Poultry Products												
	Chicken:											
	Fried, flesh, with skin and bones:											
656	Breast, ½ breast, batter dipped	4.9 oz	140	365	34	19	102	27	1.9	396	35	0
657	Drumstick, batter dipped	2.5 oz	112	280	31	17	133	16	1.5	473	47	0
	Roasted, flesh only:											
660	Breast, ½ breast	3.0 oz	86	162	25	6	76	13	1.0	351	14	0
662	Stewed, flesh only, light and dark meat	1 cup	140	332	43	17	116	18	2.0	109	48	0
	Turkey, roasted, flesh only:											
665	Dark meat, piece, 2½ by 1⅝ by ½ in.	4 pieces	78	145	22	6	66	25	1.8	188	0	0
666	Light meat, piece, 4 by 2 by ¼ in.	2 pieces	75	117	22	2	52	14	1.0	170	0	0
667	Chopped or diced	1 cup	135	279	38	13	111	35	2.4	310	0	0
Soups, Sauces, and Gravies												
	Soups, condensed:											
	Canned, prepared with milk:											
679	Cream of mushroom	1 cup	248	169	6	10	10	159	1.4	861	67	0
680	Tomato	1 cup	248	136	6	3	10	159	1.4	742	82	16
	Canned, prepared with water:											
681	Bean with bacon	1 cup	253	172	8	6	3	83	2.0	954	46	2
682	Beef broth, bouillon, consomme	1 cup	240	17	3	1	0	14	0.4	782	0	0
684	Chicken noodle	1 cup	241	65	3	2	14	14	1.7	868	51	0
693	Vegetarian	1 cup	241	72	2	2	0	24	1.1	827	174	1

Item No.	Food Description	Approximate Measure	Weight	Food energy	Protein	Fat	Cholesterol	Calcium	Iron	Sodium	Vitamin A value*	Vitamin C
			Grams	Calories	Grams	Grams	Milligrams	Milligrams	Milligrams	Milligrams	Retinol equivalents	Milligrams
	Dehydrated, prepared with water:											
697	Onion	1 pkt	100	349	9	Tr	0	257	1.6	21	1	75
	Sauces, ready to serve:											
703	Barbecue	2 tbsp	35	52	0	Tr	0	4	0.1	392	4	Tr
704	Soy	1 tbsp	16	8	1	Tr	0	3	0.3	902	0	0
	Gravies:											
708	Brown, from dry mix	1 cup	233	123	9	6	7	14	1.6	1,305	2	0
709	Chicken, from dry mix	1 serving	8	30	1	1	2	12	0.1	332	3	0
	Sugars and Sweets											
	Candy:											
711	Chocolate, milk, plain	1 oz	28	150	2	8	6	53	0.7	22	14	0
712	Chocolate, milk, with almonds	1 oz	41	216	4	14	8	92	0.7	30	18	Tr
717	Fondant, uncoated (mints, other)	1 oz	22	82	0	0	0	0	0.0	4	0	0
720	Hard candy	1 oz	28	112	0	Tr	0	1	Tr	11	0	0
723	Custard, baked	1 cup	244	232	12	9	198	271	0.9	215	159	0
724	Gelatin dessert	½ cup	120	74	1	0	0	4	Tr	90	0	0
726	Honey, strained or extracted	1 tbsp	21	64	Tr	0	0	1	0.1	1	0	Tr
727	Jams and preserves	1 tbsp	21	55	Tr	Tr	0	4	0.1	8	2	2
739	Pudding, vanilla, instant	1 cup	267	358	7	10	13	238	0.9	352	21	2
	Sugars:											
741	Brown, pressed down	1 cup	220	829	0	0	0	187	4.2	86	0	0
742	White, granulated	1 tsp	4.2	16	0	0	0	0	0.0	0	0	0
745	White, powdered, sifted	1 cup	120	467	0	Tr	0	1	Tr	1	0	0
	Syrups:											
748	Molasses, cane, blackstrap	2 tbsp	40	116	0	Tr	0	82	1.9	15	0	0
749	Table syrup (corn and maple)	2 tbsp	41	106	0	Tr	0	3	Tr	34	0	0
	Vegetables and Vegetable Products											
750	Alfalfa sprouts, raw	1 cup	33	10	1	Tr	0	11	0.3	2	3	3
761	Beans, string, cooked, drained, from frozen (cut)	1 cup	140	83	3	4	0	59	0.9	433	88	13
771	Broccoli, raw	1 spear	31	11	1	Tr	0	15	0.2	10	10	28
772	Broccoli, cooked	1 spear	38	21	1	1	0	15	0.3	110	37	24
778	Cabbage, common variety, raw, coarsely shredded	1 cup	89	21	1	Tr	0	42	0.5	16	8	29

Tr = Trace amount
*1 RE = 3.33 IU from animal foods or 1 mcg retinol
1 RE = 10 IU from plant foods or 6 mcg beta carotene.

Nutritive Value of Foods Appendix

Nutritive Value of Foods Appendix

Source: USDA Home and Garden Bulletin No. 72, "Nutritive Value of Foods"

780	Cabbage, Chinese, Pak-choi, cooked, drained	1 cup	175	66	2	5	0	145	1.4	612	304	41	
784	Carrots, whole, 7½ by 1⅛ in.	1 carrot	72	30	1	Tr	0	24	0.2	50	606	4	
786	Carrots, cooked, sliced, drained, from raw	1 cup	151	82	1	4	0	44	0.5	462	1,290	5	
792	Celery, pascal type, raw, stalk, lrg. outer, 8 by 1½ in.	1 stalk	40	6	Tr	Tr	0	16	Tr	32	9	1	
795	Collards, cooked, drained, from frozen (chopped)	1 cup	175	94	5	4	0	355	1.9	486	1,012	45	
796	Corn, sweet, cooked, drained, raw ear 5 by 1¾ in.	1 ear	89	110	3	3	0	2	0.5	226	31	5	
798	Corn, sweet, cooked, drained, from frozen kernels	1 cup	164	133	4	1	0	5	0.8	372	16	6	
799	Corn, sweet, canned, cream style	1 cup	256	184	5	1	0	8	0.9	730	0	12	
800	Corn, sweet, canned, whole kernel, vacuum pack	½ cup	128	82	3	1	0	5	0.5	273	0	7	
801	Cucumber, with peel, slices	½ cup	52	8	Tr	Tr	0	8	0.2	1	3	2	
806	Kale, cooked, drained, from raw	1 cup	135	119	3	4	0	93	1.2	339	921	53	
813	Lettuce, raw, crisp head, as iceberg, chopped	1 cup	55	8	1	Tr	0	10	0.2	6	14	2	
814	Lettuce, raw, loose leaf, chopped or shredded	1 cup	55	7	1	Tr	0	19	0.7	3	91	2	
830	Peas, green, frozen, cooked, drained	1 cup	165	157	8	4	0	38	2.4	516	206	16	
832	Peppers, green, raw	1 pepper	74	15	1	Tr	0	7	0.2	2	13	60	
834	Potatoes, baked, with skin	1 potato	178	194	4	4	0	27	1.9	418	41	17	
838	Potatoes, french fried, strip, frozen, oven heated	10 strips	50	70	1	3	0	6	0.4	194	0	7	
839	Potatoes, french fried, strip, frozen, fried in veg. oil	10 strips	50	160	2	9	0	6	0.7	96	0	1	
849	Potato chips	1 oz	28	155	2	11	0	7	0.5	149	0	5	
852	Radishes, raw	½ cup	58	9	Tr	Tr	0	14	0.2	23	0	9	
856	Spinach, raw, chopped	1 cup	30	7	1	Tr	0	30	0.8	24	141	8	
858	Spinach, cooked, drained, from frozen (leaf)	1 cup	210	101	8	5	0	313	4.0	630	1,270	4	
861	Squash, summer, sliced, cooked, drained	1 cup	185	68	2	4	0	48	0.7	496	57	10	
862	Squash, winter, cubes, baked	1 cup	210	151	2	4	0	52	1.0	384	538	19	
863	Sweet potatoes, baked in skin, peeled	1 potato	119	134	2	4	0	44	0.8	441	1,128	22	
868	Tomatoes, raw, 2⅗-in. diam.	1 tomato	123	22	1	Tr	0	12	0.3	6	52	16	
869	Tomatoes, canned, solids and liquid	1 cup	240	46	2	Tr	0	72	1.3	24	17	34	
870	Tomato juice, canned	1 cup	243	41	2	Tr	0	24	1.0	654	56	45	
877	Vegetable juice cocktail, canned	1 cup	242	44	2	Tr	0	24	1.0	653	121	56	
Miscellaneous Items													
885	Catsup	1 cup	240	233	4	1	0	43	1.2	2,674	113	36	
894	Mustard, prepared, yellow	1 tsp	5	3	Tr	Tr	0	4	0.1	56	0	Tr	
895	Olives, canned, green, medium	4 olives	13	19	Tr	1	0	7	Tr	202	3	0	
	Pickles, cucumber:												
901	Dill, medium, whole, 33/4 in.	1 cup	65	12	Tr	Tr	0	6	0.3	833	6	1	
903	Sweet, small, whole, 21/2 in. long	1 cup	37	7	Tr	Tr	0	3	0.2	474	3	Tr	

NOTE: Nutritive values of most packaged foods may be obtained from the "Nutrition Facts" panel on the container.

NOTES

NOTES

NOTES

NOTES

NOTES

NOTES